P9-BZS-024

The Complete Idiot's Reference Card

A Little Heart-Healthy Effort Goes a Long Way

It doesn't take much to keep your heart healthy and happy. It's as easy as one, two, three to lower your blood pressure and blood cholesterol levels:

1. Don't smoke. (If you do smoke, quit.)
2. Exercise 30 minutes most days.
3. Lower the amount of fat in your diet.

Your Heart-Healthy Lifestyle

While everyone can benefit from the basic guidelines for heart health, each of us has different circumstances and needs. In what ways can you change your lifestyle to make your heart healthy and happy?

Current Behavior	Heart-Healthy Replacement
1. Eat too much ice cream	1. Fat-free sorbet _____
2. Ignore regular check-ups	2. Schedule annual physicals
3. Too much sitting at work	3. Take a walk during lunch hour
4. _____	4. _____
5. _____	5. _____
6. _____	6. _____
7. _____	7. _____
8. _____	8. _____
9. _____	9. _____
10. _____	10. _____

alpha
books

CPR for Adults

You can't learn CPR by just reading about it!

If you haven't taken a CPR class, make it a priority to sign up for one. Keep this card in a safe place as a reminder of the basic steps for this life-saving procedure.

First, if other people are around, shout "Heart attack!" and ask for someone to call for emergency aid (usually 911 in the United States). Make sure the person is in cardiac arrest. Check for signs of breathing and a pulse.

To begin CPR, follow these steps:

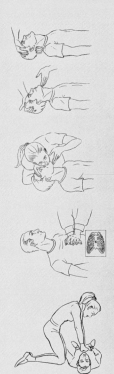

- ➤ Place the person on his or her back on a hard, flat surface (the floor is ideal).

- ➤ Tip the head back so the chin juts up (the mouth should fall open).

- ➤ Pinch the nose shut, take a deep breath, place your mouth over the victim's mouth, and blow.

- ➤ Wait 10 seconds to see if the person begins breathing. If not, give another breath and then begin cardiac compressions.

- ➤ Place the heel of your hand in the middle of the breastbone, then place the heel of your other hand over the back of your hand.

- ➤ Lock your elbows to keep your arms straight. Press down quickly and forcefully so the breastbone depresses $1^{1}/_{2}$ to 2 inches, then release.

- ➤ Do this at a rate of 80 compressions per minute if you are alone, giving two breaths after every 15 compressions. If there are two of you, one should do the breathing and other the compressions at a rate of one breath every five compressions.

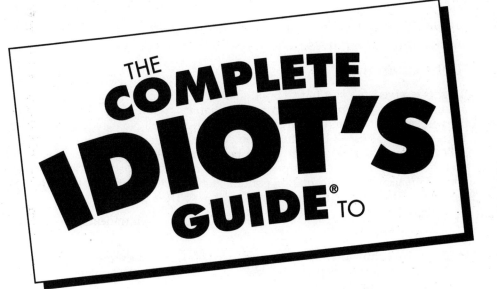

THE COMPLETE IDIOT'S GUIDE® TO

a Happy, Healthy Heart

*by Deborah S. Romaine
and Dawn E. DeWitt, M.D.*

alpha books

A Division of Macmillan General Reference
A Simon & Schuster Macmillan Company
1633 Broadway, New York, NY 10019-6785

For our children, may we teach them heart-healthy habits to carry them through long, happy lives.

©1998 Amaranth

All rights reserved. No part of this book shall be reproduced, stored in a retrieval system, or transmitted by any means, electronic, mechanical, photocopying, recording, or otherwise, without written permission from the publisher. No patent liability is assumed with respect to the use of the information contained herein. Although every precaution has been taken in the preparation of this book, the publisher and authors assume no responsibility for errors or omissions. Neither is any liability assumed for damages resulting from the use of the information contained herein. For information, address Alpha Books, 1633 Broadway, 7th Floor, New York, NY 10019-6785.

THE COMPLETE IDIOT'S GUIDE TO & Design is a registered trademarks of Prentice-Hall, Inc.

Macmillan Publishing books may be purchased for business or sales promotional use. For information please write: Special Markets Department, Macmillan Publishing USA, 1633 Broadway, New York, NY 10019.

International Standard Book Number 0-02-862393-2

Library of Congress Catalog Card Number: 98-86098

00 99 98   8 7 6 5 4 3 2 1

Interpretation of the printing code: the rightmost number of the first series of numbers is the year of the book's printing; the rightmost number of the second series of numbers is the number of the book's printing. For example, a printing code of 98-1 shows that the first printing of the book occurred in 1998.

Printed in the United States of America

Note: This publication contains the opinions and ideas of its authors. It is intended to provide helpful and informative material on the subject matter covered. It is sold with the understanding that the authors and publisher are not engaged in rendering professional services in the book. If the reader requires personal assistance or advice, a competent professional should be consulted.

The authors and publisher specifically disclaim any responsibility for any liability, loss or risk, personal or otherwise, which is incurred as a consequence, directly or indirectly, of the use and application of any of the contents of this book.

Alpha Development Team

Publisher
Kathy Nebenhaus

Editorial Director
Gary M. Krebs

Managing Editor
Bob Shuman

Marketing Brand Manager
Felice Primeau

Senior Editor
Nancy Mikhail

Development Editors
Phil Kitchel
Jennifer Perillo
Amy Zavatto

Editorial Assistant
Maureen Horn

Production Team

Book Producer
Lee Ann Chearney, Amaranth

Development Editor
Matthew X. Kiernan

Production Editor
Donna Wright

Copy Editor
Fran Blauw

Cover Designer
Mike Freeland

Photo Editor
Richard H. Fox

Cartoonist
Jody P. Schaeffer

Illustrator
David McGrievey

Designer
Glenn Larsen

Indexer
Chris Barrick

Layout/Proofreading
Angela Calvert
Kim Cofer
Pamela Woolf

3399

Contents at a Glance

Contents

Part 6: Putting Your Heart in the Right Place 239

Foreword

An old Latin proverb says *Mens sana in corpore sano,* meaning "healthy mind in a healthy body." George Bernard Shaw echoes, "The sound body is a product of the sound mind."

In my view, body and mind are intrinsically connected and mutually conditioned. Therefore, a more holistic approach to the care of the individual would attend to the needs of the body, of the heart, as well as the quests of the spirit. We are witnessing a profound transformation in the history of medicine: the old doctor-centered medicine yields to the modern patient-centered medicine. A new triad emerges: a closer patient-physician relationship, patient's education, and patient's empowerment. Empowered patients are less likely to succumb to illness.

This book offers you a compendium of modern scientific knowledge. Clear text and illustrations facilitate the understanding of complex issues, and fundamental concepts are crystallized at the end of each chapter. Valuable tools for self-assessment will provide you a key to some critical lifestyle changes and to a more spiritual dimension of health. As your mind progressively conquers peace through self-awareness and meditation, your heart rests and rejuvenates itself.

In the pathway toward self-mastering, toward a happy, healthy heart, you will feel pervaded by a wave of optimistic realism and uplifting hope and become motivated to achieve higher levels of physical, mental, and spiritual well-being. In your newly found harmony of body and spirit will reside the power of self-healing.

—Bruno S. Cortis, M.D.

Dr. Cortis is a board-certified internist, a practicing cardiologist, a pioneer in angioplasty and laser applications, and the founder of the Exceptional Heart Patients Program in Illinois. He is the author of *Heart and Soul,* a psychological and spiritual guide to preventing and healing heart disease.

Introduction

How's your heart today? Have you ever worried about having heart problems? Has your doctor told you to be careful? Do heart problems run in your family? Is your heart a bit heavy, maybe even overworked? Then you're in the right place! By picking up this book, you've made the first of what we hope will be many heart-healthy choices.

It's amazingly easy to be careless with your lifestyle, even when you know what's heart-healthy and what's a fast track to an early grave. As long as you seem to have no problems, it's easy to believe that you never will. Which, of course, couldn't be further from the truth!

As busy professionals and working parents ourselves, we know firsthand the pressures of juggling priorities. We know it's not always easy to eat right and exercise regularly; life is sometimes more about squeezing minutes from the hour than hours from the day. We've tried to carry this understanding through in our writing and to suggest ways that you can make the most of the opportunities you have. As you read, we want you to feel like you're having a nice talk with your doctor, the kind of chat doctors don't often have time for during office visits. And we hope that if you have questions about your heart health, you'll take them to your doctor for answers that could save your life.

How to Use This Book

There's no right way to eat an apple, and there's no absolute way to read this book. You don't have to read it all at once, or even in order, though certainly you can do either. We've organized this book into six parts, each presenting a different aspect of heart health. You can skip right to the part that interests you most, or start at the beginning and build your understanding and knowledge layer by layer. Self-tests throughout provide you with humorous insights into your present lifestyle choices. Each chapter ends with a few key messages in a short summary called "The Least You Need to Know."

Part 1, "Health Is Where the Heart Is," introduces the basics: what makes your heart tick, what your heart needs to make it happy, and what role you have in shaping your heart's health and happiness.

Part 2, "How Do You Mend a 'Broken' Heart?," looks at what can go wrong with your heart and what modern medical technology offers in the way of fixing your heart problems.

Part 3, "The Way to Heart Health Is Through Your Stomach," explores the relationship between what crosses your lips and your heart's health. Learn what's wrong with our typical eating habits and how to change yours for the good of your heart.

Part 4, "Exercise Makes the Heart Grow Stronger," investigates how physical activity affects the health of your heart. Are your sedentary ways leading you to an early grave?

Part 5, "Change Is the Law of Life," looks at how you live and what risky choices you make. There's more truth to the adage "live fast, die young" than you might realize.

Part 6, "Putting Your Heart in the Right Place," returns to the body/mind connection, exploring ways to strengthen this bond for the health and happiness of both.

Heart Hints

Sprinkled throughout are tidbits of information you might find interesting or helpful, set aside in boxes.

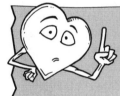

Take It to Heart

Here, you'll get information that supplements material in the text, like bits of history and interesting stories.

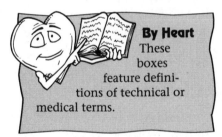

By Heart
These boxes feature definitions of technical or medical terms.

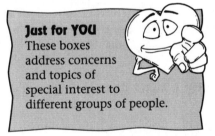

Just for YOU
These boxes address concerns and topics of special interest to different groups of people.

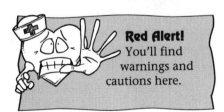

Red Alert!
You'll find warnings and cautions here.

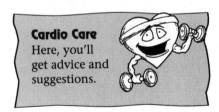

Cardio Care
Here, you'll get advice and suggestions.

Trademarks

Terms suspected of being trademarks or service marks have been appropriately capitalized. Alpha Books cannot attest to the accuracy of this information. Use of a term in this book should not be regarded as affecting the validity of any trademark or service mark.

Acknowledgments

Never is it possible to thank all the people who make a book happen, but always we try. We thank... The colleagues who shared opinions and advice. The librarians who so cheerfully and efficiently handled our requests for information and materials. The friends who put up with our total immersion in our writing. And especially, we thank our families. In particular, Debbie thanks Mike, who's had the tolerance of a saint; Chris and Cassidy; who handled their mother's temporary insanity with maturity beyond their years; Denise and Ava, with their uncanny ability to call in times of need; and John, Joyce, Leon, Lonna, and Reba for their support and understanding. Dawn extends her special thanks to Alan, who let her work on the computer late into the night; Doug and Steve, colleagues who got her started on the adventures of teaching and writing; and her patients, who've taught her about being a good doctor. We both give our heartfelt gratitude to Lee Ann Chearney at Amaranth, our book producer, who always offered just the right blend of encouragement and enthusiasm. Lastly, we dedicate this book to loved ones we've lost to heart disease—Debbie her father, and Dawn the grandfather who cared about every detail of her doctor-progress and who would be pleased as punch to read this book.

Special Thanks to Our Technical Reviewer

The Complete Idiot's Guide to a Happy, Healthy Heart was reviewed by an expert who double-checked the accuracy of what you'll learn here, to help us ensure that this book gives you everything you need to know about a happy, healthy heart. Special thanks are extended to Steven J. Compton, M.D., FACC, for his expert technical review of this book. A cardiology specialist who trained at the University of Washington in Seattle, Dr. Compton directs the Noninvasive Cardiology Laboratory and teaches at the University of Utah Health Science Center in Salt Lake City, Utah. A great skier, world traveler, and pilot, Dr. Compton balances a healthy lifestyle with an awesome ability to take care of sick hearts.

Part 1
Health Is Where the Heart Is

*"What the arms do, where the legs take us, how all the parts of the body move—
all of this the heart ordains."*

—ancient Egyptian saying

*So what is this living pump that beats, rhythmically and automatically, deep within
your chest? The ancient Egyptians weren't so far off—your heart gives the rest of your
body its marching orders. This miracle muscle propels you through a lifetime of days
and nights, seemingly without effort or variation. Don't be fooled. Your heart needs
your help to keep your body healthy.*

*The chapters in Part 1 take you on a tour of the human heart, from the perceptions of
ancient cultures to the knowledge of modern science. Come on in—what you learn
could change (and lengthen) your life!*

Chapter 1

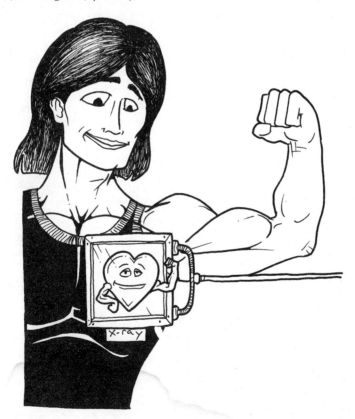

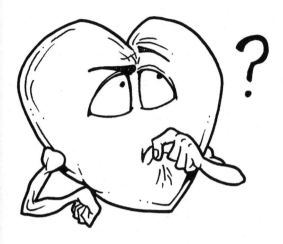

What Makes a Heart Happy and Healthy?

In This Chapter

➤ A history of the heart

➤ Lifestyle choices for a happy, healthy heart

➤ Why diet and exercise is important

➤ Your personal pursuit of happiness

"How are you?" we casually ask each other. Do you automatically answer, "Fine," without thinking much about it? Most people do. There just isn't time to share the details of our daily lives. Every day, from dawn to dusk and often deep into the night, we're on the move, taking care of the business of living. With so many things to do, so many responsibilities, so many challenges, our lives often seem to move us, sweeping us from one moment to the next and one place to the next.

While our minds focus on the events that propel our lives, our hearts beat out the rhythm of vitality that drives life itself. We don't usually think much about this muscle that is our life force. Like a good movie score, the beating heart is just there, paralleling the action in our lives. When deadlines and schedules stress our minds, our hearts race. When we tenderly tuck our children in at night, our hearts are calm and steady.

If you ask your heart, "How are you?" how would it answer? What makes a heart happy and healthy?

On the Motion of the Heart and Blood

Is the heart merely a mechanical pump that keeps the body alive? Or is it the center of our emotions, our soul and sense of well-being? From the dawn of human civilization, the beating in our chests has been both the voice of life and the sound of comfort. Ancient cave paintings show that prehistoric cultures viewed the heart as an animating force, a timekeeper, and a comforter. The mother who draws her fussy baby to her breast knows the strong and familiar rhythm of her heartbeat will soothe her child. Her simple, "instinctive" action stretches across eons of time to connect her with other mothers who once did the same thing. For all the scientific advancements that mark our time, the beating heart remains for us what it was for prehistoric cultures—the source of life and solace.

Since the earliest times, humankind has yearned to know more about this beating heart. Early efforts to understand the mysteries of the heart and circulatory system combined physical discoveries with spiritual beliefs. The most practiced ancient Egyptian physicians could "hear" the body "tell" of its ailments through the voice of the heart by placing their fingers on pulse points in the arms, legs, neck, and torso. They no doubt learned to connect changes in the heart rate, or pulse, with certain disease conditions. (If you sit still and concentrate on your heartbeat, you'll quickly become aware of the pulsing motion of blood through your body.) These same practitioners also regarded the heart as the "seat of the mind" and left it in a body being prepared for burial, believing that the heart's weight would help the gods determine the soul's new existence in its next life.

By Heart

Meta-physics means "after the physical," an apt description for studies that examine what is beyond objective observation. The ancient Greeks used meta-physics to explore the functions of the human body they could not directly observe, as well as humankind's place in the universe. As a result of his investigations, Greek philosopher Aristotle concluded that the heart was the most important organ in the body and the center of intelligence.

The religious beliefs the ancient Egyptians attached to the heart kept them from cutting it open to see how it was constructed. Early Greek physicians learned much about anatomy from treating battle wounds that exposed internal organs, though they lacked the means to investigate how the body's systems worked. Taking a more holistic approach, early Chinese physicians viewed the body's organs as an inseparable combination of structure and function. While they wrote about the circular flow of blood based on what they could feel, they didn't know how this flow sustained life.

That the heart was essential to life, however, went undisputed. Across cultures and ages, the organ continued to be described metaphysically as the center of human emotions. Ancient Greek scholars, such as Empedocles and Hippocrates, used philosophy to explain what they could not observe about the role of the heart.

Take It to Heart

The heart and the circulation of the blood have long been central to healers and healing. Empedocles (490–430 B.C.) wrote, "The blood around men's heart is their thinking." He believed the four elements of the physical world—air, earth, water, and fire—were most thoroughly mixed in the blood, making the blood the source of thought. Hippocrates (460–377 B.C., often called the Father of Medicine, emphasized the relationship between the whole body and its parts. Shortly before Hippocrates died, the man who would become known as the Father of Anatomy, Herophilus, was born. The first to measure pulse rate, Herophilus developed an elaborate treatment scheme based on "letting blood" in affected body parts to heal them by restoring balance to the blood.

For several hundred years, antediluvian medical practice focused on achieving balance among the four humors that Hippocrates defined as the essence of life—yellow bile, black bile, blood, and phlegm—to treat everything from asthma to warts. Hippocrates was also the first to identify the brain, not the heart, as the center of consciousness, though this concept took a while longer to catch on. Over the centuries, the Greeks learned more about the heart, most notably through the discoveries of the physician Galen (A.D. 130–200), who used the pulse to make medical diagnoses. While Galen was the first Western physician to correctly connect the functions of the lungs, heart, arteries, and veins in their roles of transporting oxygen and removing waste, his understanding of the human circulatory system was complex and not quite accurate. Based on his observations, Galen incorrectly concluded that the liver was the center of the circulatory system and that the veins that came from it sent nutrients to the body's vital organs. The arteries, Galen said, carried "vital spirits" from the heart to the rest of the body.

Medical practitioners followed Galen's ideas until the Renaissance. In this era of discovery, the brilliant Italian scientist and artist Leonardo da Vinci (1452–1519) and, after him, the Belgian anatomist Andreas Vesalius (1514–64) began to produce drawings of the body based on dissections of cadavers, which changed the world's understanding of the human heart.

English physician William Harvey (1578–1657) proved that the mechanical pumping action of the heart muscle circulates blood throughout the body, with the arteries carrying it away from the heart and the veins returning it. Harvey's book, *On the Motion of the Heart and Blood,* published in 1628, presented Harvey's radical redefinition of the body's circulatory system and established him as the Father of Modern Physiology.

In our own century, we've made discoveries about the heart that are just as profound. On December 3, 1967, South African surgeon Christiaan Barnard performed the first successful human heart transplant operation. In December 1982, William C. DeVries, an American, implanted an artificial heart designed by Robert Jarvik into patient Dr. Barney Clark, who lived 112 days. Yet our extensive state-of-the-art knowledge of the heart as a pumping engine that powers the human "machine" still exists hand in hand with an overwhelming conviction by many physicians, psychologists, and laypersons that emotional states and the body are joined—though precisely how and where they are joined remains unclear. Increasingly, physicians are considering the emotions and lifestyles of patients as important factors in understanding and treating illness as well as in fostering wellness.

While Harvey was working on a new view of the physical heart, the English poet and playwright William Shakespeare (1564–1616) was creating masterpieces of the emotional "heart." Plays including *Hamlet, Romeo and Juliet,* and *A Midsummer Night's Dream* were published in collected form in 1623 as the now famous First Folio, only five years before Harvey's scientific classic revolutionized medical thinking of the time. What a fantastic synchronicity of two achievements that so dramatically advanced our understanding of the human heart!

The heart remains for our generation a vital metaphor for what it means to be human, just as it was for cave painters in prehistoric times and for artists throughout the ages, such as Leonardo da Vinci, Shakespeare, and others. Our unique 21st-century perspective allows us to investigate this metaphor using sophisticated technology unavailable to earlier artists.

Russian-American dancer and choreographer Mikhail Baryshnikov blends art and science to explore the body/mind connection in a very personal way. In his performance "Heart-beat: MB," Baryshnikov attaches a wireless device to his chest while he dances to amplify electrical impulses from his brain to his heart and muscles. "You're totally transparent," Baryshnikov says of the experience in an interview with the *New York Times.* "Your heart is very much connected to your mind. And that is what this piece is about, in general: the heart as a pumping instrument and the heart as all the old clichés about the heart, from ancient poetry to the modern medical tracts."

What Comes From the Heart, Goes to the Heart

"What comes from the heart, goes to the heart." The 19th-century English Romantic poet Samuel Taylor Coleridge may have been writing about human emotions when he penned these words, but there's more than a little scientific truth to them as well. How long do you think it takes for the heart to send one drop of blood, purified by the lungs, on a complete circuit of your body? An average of 24 seconds! That means one drop of blood circulates through your body about 3,600 times a day.

Without the continuous pumping action of your heart, your body would die almost immediately. That's a fact you live with every day and probably don't think much about—that is, until something begins to go wrong. Maybe we should think about it. According to the American Heart Association, nearly 60 million Americans have one or more forms of *cardiovascular disease* (CVD). CVD is the single leading cause of death in America today.

Clearly, we need to pay more attention to our hearts. And that means paying more attention to the way we live our lives. How are you? How do you feel today? Do you find yourself too often tired, unable to concentrate, frustrated, short of breath after even the smallest amount of physical exertion? Are you harried and stressed out? Is it impossible to keep up with your life, much less feel like you're getting ahead? Do you grab whatever's quick and easy to eat, without thinking about what exactly you're putting into your body or whether you're enjoying it?

We assume our hearts and our bodies are strong enough to take whatever treatment we give them and still thrive. And why not? The average life span in 1998 is about 75 years, almost double the 45-year average American life span in 1900. Medical technology is on our side. If something goes wrong, we can just take a pill or get a doctor to come in and "fix" it. We live in a time like no other in the history of humankind, a time when new drugs, therapies, and treatments can actually repair, and often restore, damaged hearts to health. These are certainly remarkable and wonderful developments.

Do we really enhance our lives or our health if we depend on these medical advances to bail us out, to save us from taking responsibility for the choices we make each day? As the saying goes, "What goes around, comes around." Not every case of heart disease can be reversed or prevented. But a strong heart is in better shape to handle problems that might develop. We can make choices that not only promote the health of our hearts and entire cardiovascular systems, but enrich the "heart" of our life experiences as well.

You get the point. If you take care of your heart, your heart will take care of you. It's that simple—and that difficult. In the heat of the moment, it's sometimes hard to ask yourself, "Is what I'm doing good for my health and my heart?" Too many times, we decide that just this one time, it won't hurt. But that one time becomes another, and before you know it, what you're doing is a way of life. A million Americans lose their lives each year to heart disease. That's 700 to 1,000 deaths a day.

By Heart

Cardiovascular comes from the Greek word *kardia,* which means "heart," and the Latin word *vasculum,* which means "small vessel," referring to blood vessels. *Cardiovascular disease* (CVD) consists of high blood pressure, coronary heart disease, stroke, rheumatic heart disease, and other heart and blood vessel problems.

Just for YOU

Do you take medication for high blood pressure, high blood cholesterol, and other heart problems? Doctors write more than 157 million prescriptions a year for such drugs, making them the third most commonly prescribed medications (behind pain relief and antibiotics) in the United States. Don't let your "fast fix" lull you into thinking you're now "covered" for indulgences, though. Heart healthy lifestyle changes can keep you from being just another statistic.

Do you see yourself in any of these situations?

> **Red Alert!**
> Do you have:
> pressure or
> pain in the chest
> lasting more than a few
> minutes; pain in the shoulder,
> neck, or arms; and chest
> discomfort with lightheaded-
> ness, fainting, sweating,
> nausea, or shortness of breath?
> If these symptoms last longer
> than 15 or 20 minutes or
> happen during exercise, you
> may be having a heart attack.
> Minutes count—get medical
> attention immediately!

➤ You'd rather reach for the remote control and sit for hours in front of the TV than take a brisk walk around your neighborhood.

➤ You opt for that fourth cup of coffee and gulp down a candy bar at the office for some quick afternoon energy, leaving you full of empty calories, unable to get to sleep at night and tired the next morning.

➤ Steps? You take the elevator or escalator every time. And walking? Forget it. Cars are for getting from one place to another.

➤ Stress? You believe that's just an inevitable fact of modern life, and any time you try to have a less stressful life, it just creates more stress. The stress you have already is just fine, thank you!

➤ Heart trouble runs in your family, so there's nothing you can do about it. You might as well live it up while you're still healthy.

➤ You'd consider changing your diet to make it more healthful—as long as you don't have to give up steak, eggs, or cheese.

➤ You know you should stop smoking. Everyone in America knows it. You'll do it; you'll stop tomorrow (or next week, or next month…).

Well, we know you're no idiot. You're reading this book because you want to have a happy, healthy heart. And you don't have to wait until you find yourself a guest star at your local hospital's ER (that's *emergency room…*) to decide to start living heart healthy. You can start doing the things your heart needs to be healthy and happy right now, today! It's all a matter of choice.

What the Heart Needs

Go to any primary care physician or cardiologist and ask what a happy, healthy heart needs. (By the way, when was your last checkup?) Chances are, you already know in your heart (pun intended) what you'll hear. That's right: diet, exercise, no smoking, and stress reduction. Not necessarily easy (or fun, depending on how you look at it) stuff, but definitely the right stuff.

It's good to establish an ongoing relationship with your primary care doctor. The more he or she gets to know about you, and vice versa, the better. Your primary care physician can help you prevent heart problems, treat a wide variety of heart conditions, or may refer you to a physician who specializes in heart problems called a *cardiologist*. Cardiologists typically see patients only by referral. Many health insurance programs, especially managed care programs such as HMOs, require a referral from a primary care physician before they will pay for care provided by a cardiologist.

The real challenge: How do you come up with a heart-healthy program that makes you happy? That is, one that you—and your heart—can live with. It may not be as difficult as it seems at first glance. Sure, the optimum heart-healthy program would have you on a diet with only 10 to 15 percent of calories from fat. You'd be making exercise an everyday part of your life. You'd never smoke another cigarette. You'd sign up for a stress-reduction program or a class in meditation or yoga. But, hey, one thing at a time is better than nothing. In this century of instant gratification, we think we have to be able to accomplish something in the blink of an eye to be successful. That's not true. Work with your physician to find out where you are on the heart-healthy spectrum and start from there. Make small moves, set small goals, and stick to them—take it one day at a time.

Eating Heart Smart

We all need to think about and strive for a good diet. In the United States, where our cultural norm is a high-fat diet full of processed, chemical-filled, sugar-laden convenience foods, eating right can take some effort. A heart-healthy diet, in general terms, is low in fat, reduces your overall cholesterol level, and improves your ratio of "good" and "bad" cholesterol. (More on this in Part 3, "The Way to Heart Health Is Through Your Stomach.") Also, controlling your weight reduces the risk of heart disease. The more you weigh, the higher your risk. If you've been struggling with a weight problem for years, heart health may be just the motivation you need to take off those extra pounds.

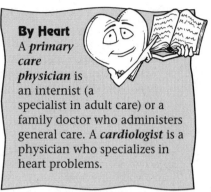

By Heart
A *primary care physician* is an internist (a specialist in adult care) or a family doctor who administers general care. A *cardiologist* is a physician who specializes in heart problems.

Cardio Care
In our instant gratification culture, we've come to expect results in the blink of an eye. Television and movies resolve conflicts and crises between commercials. Real life doesn't work that way. There is no recipe for an instant healthy heart. In most people, heart disease takes decades to develop. So the earlier you make heart-healthy lifestyle changes, the happier your heart will be...and stay.

If you don't know a lot about nutrition, now's the time to start learning. In a recent telephone survey, 70 percent of the people who participated believed they had healthy diet habits—yet the diets they described were much too high in fat and much too low in fresh vegetables and fruits, legumes (beans to you and me), and grains. Don't make any assumptions about how healthy your current diet is. Do the research on good nutrition. Then, compare how your diet stacks up. What about your diet do you need to change? How can you adopt heart-healthy menus featuring dishes you'll actually want to eat? (In Part 3, we'll give you strategies that will make the process easier.)

What the Heart Doesn't Need: Couch Potatoes

According to the American College of Physicians, only 22 percent of American adults are active enough right now to benefit health-wise. In a report to encourage doctors to help patients become more active, the ACP asserts, "Inactive persons who improve their physical fitness are less likely to die of all causes and of cardiovascular disease than those who are sedentary." The bottom line? Get up and start moving around. Take a walk. Take the stairs. March in place. Ride a bike. Anything that puts your body in motion. Just get moving!

Not the type who goes to gyms? Never going to let anyone see you in a pair of shorts, much less in an aerobics class? Always the last one picked in PE class in school? Forget it! Anyone can become physically fit. And if your goal is to lose weight as well as improve your fitness level, there's no better decision you can make than to start exercising. We have this to say to anyone reading this book who is shy or intimidated about beginning an exercise program: Everyone has to start somewhere! (Even Jane Fonda and Arnold Schwarzenegger had to start somewhere.)

Whenever you're about to begin a new exercise program, consult your physician for advice on the best choices for your individual needs. Consider bringing in a personal trainer to work with you, at least in the beginning. Look for a trainer who has graduated from an educational program in exercise physiology.

Improving your fitness level is the best gift you can give to yourself and to your heart. And you can do it by engaging in 30 minutes of moderately intense activity each day. Mow the lawn, take the stairs instead of the elevator, treat yourself to a daily walk of three or so miles. Still sound like a lot? Okay, make it your goal, and work up to it. Already pretty fit? Reward yourself with an extra round of your favorite activity, and remember that there's always room for improvement. Exercising engages us in life's events. It brings us into contact with other people and the world around us in vital, exciting ways. You might like it more than you expect. (Find out more about exercise and your heart in Part 4, "Exercise Makes the Heart Grow Stronger.")

> **Cardio Care**
> Think exercise programs are too expensive? Medical studies prove that exercise adds years to your life. What else could be a better value for the money?

Breaking Bad Habits

You've heard about the studies: A drink a day is healthy for your heart. So should you drink alcohol? Let's put it this way: If you don't drink now, don't start. The risks of alcohol very probably outweigh the questionable benefits to your heart. If you do drink, remember that alcohol contributes nothing nutritionally for the calories it adds to your daily intake. If you're worried about whether you drink too much, talk with your primary care physician.

On the subject of smoking, we have only one thing to say: Don't. The medical research is clear and overwhelming. Cigarette smoking is a major cause of heart attacks. The risks from smoking are so palpable that the Surgeon General has called smoking "the most important of known modifiable risk factors for coronary heart disease in the United States." Smoking also increases your risk of lung cancer and other cancers. The risks of secondhand smoke may be no less serious; initial studies estimate that nearly 40,000 people die each year from heart and blood vessel disease caused by environmental tobacco smoke. If you smoke now, stop. Smoking is a tremendously difficult addiction to break. But you have all the incentive to try with a happy, healthy heart as your goal.

Today it seems there's an over-the-counter or prescription drug for whatever ails you. Drug companies are growing as fast as computer-technology companies and are taking in greater profits every year. Biotech advances promise new and exciting drug therapies in the 21st century. But we need to think about what we're doing when we automatically reach for the medicine cabinet. Mixing medications is a dangerous habit. Drug interactions can be serious, and medical research is only now beginning to understand how they can affect heart health.

And remember, alcohol and nicotine are drugs, too. Read Part 5, "Change Is the Law of Life," to learn more about alcohol and easing up if you need to, nicotine and strategies to quit smoking for good, and other drugs you take and how they may affect your heart health.

Red Alert!
Make it a habit to tell your physician every drug you take—that includes vitamins, supplements, homeopathic and naturopathic (herbal) remedies, over-the-counter medications, and prescription drugs (even birth control pills). The information may keep you from experiencing unpleasant side effects—and it may even save your life!

Happiness Depends Upon Ourselves

"Happiness depends upon ourselves," said the Greek philosopher Aristotle (384–322 B.C.). Ultimately, we alone can determine what makes our lives happy. And we alone have the power to obtain that happiness. Thomas Jefferson said it, too, in his eloquent summary establishing life, liberty, and the pursuit of happiness as the rights of all individuals. The very word *pursuit* suggests action, change, and feeling. What is the pursuit of health and healing if not the pursuit of happiness?

While researchers need to further study the effects of emotional stress on the heart, scientific evidence points to a relationship between cardiovascular disease and a high-stress lifestyle. It could be that stress keeps you from making and sticking to the tough choices you'll need to make to promote heart health. How you handle stress may make an important difference for your happy, healthy heart.

The only certainty about heart health is that we don't yet know all there is to know about this wondrous organ that sustains life. Is the heart merely a mechanical pump, or is it somehow the center of feelings and emotions? While everyone has an opinion, human-kind does not yet know all there is to know about the human heart. Any investigation into its properties—scientific or emotional—is bound to lead us on a path toward a happier, healthier life. Our goal in this book is to give you the facts about the heart as we know them today so you can use the information to plan your path. Let's get started. Destination: Your happy, healthy heart!

The Least You Need to Know

➤ Throughout history, humankind has explored the nature of the heart as both the pump that powers the body and as the center of our feelings and emotions.

➤ Proactive lifestyle changes can often prevent or reverse heart disease, which is the leading killer of Americans today.

➤ The most important ways to reduce your risk of heart disease are to quit smoking, start exercising, change your diet, and reduce stress.

➤ You have the power to make positive, long-lasting, heart-healthy changes in your life.

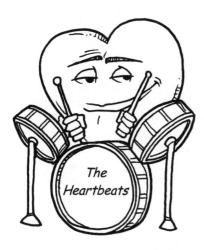

The Heartbeats

The Rhythm of Life

Tighten your right hand into a fist, then let it relax. Do this 70 or so times a minute, and you're doing a pretty good imitation of your heart in action. Now place your fist against your chest as though you were going to say the Pledge of Allegiance, just to the left of your breastbone and about four inches down from that notch you can feel at the base of your throat. Beneath your ribs, sternum, and chest muscles, your heart is hard at work. You can feel it right under your fingers!

The wondrous muscle that powers your body is about the size of your fist and weighs just under three-quarters of a pound. What you see when you look at the finger side of your clenched fist is closer to what your heart really looks like than the symmetrical shape so familiar as Cupid's trademark. Your heart begins pumping about three months after conception and can continue for 100 years or longer—about 100,000 times a day and more than 2.5 billion times during an average lifetime.

In Your Heart

The place your heart calls home is really more of a fortress, as well-protected as Fort Knox. And for good reason, because your heart holds the key to your life. The first line of defense: Those bones of Biblical fame, the ribs. Curved for extra strength, they enclose the chest in a nearly impenetrable cage. Muscles, tendons, and ligaments secure the ribs to the shield-like sternum in the front of your body and to the spine in the back. An especially strong muscle, the *diaphragm*, keeps your heart from sliding into your belly (though a good roller-coaster ride can make you feel like it does just that). A tough sac of fibrous tissue called the *pericardium* surrounds the heart, anchoring it within the chest. A thin layer of fluid flows between the sac and the heart to ease the friction that results as the heart contracts and expands.

Your heart is a model of natural efficiency. Without conscious intervention from you, it beats more than 100,000 times a day, circulating life-giving blood throughout your body.

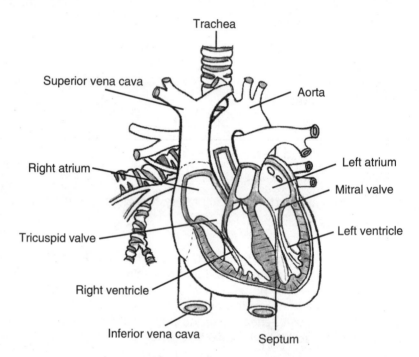

Your heart is made of *myocardium*, a strong, special kind of muscle not found anywhere else in your body. If you cut open a heart (not yours, of course!), you might be surprised to find that it's hollow inside. A thin wall of muscle called the *septum* divides your heart from top to bottom, making a left side and a right side. Each side has two chambers, or cavities—an *atrium* on the top and a *ventricle* on the bottom. The atrium functions like a waiting room, while the ventricle is where all the action takes place. A one-way valve lets blood flow from the atrium to the ventricle and prevents it from flowing back the other way.

The hard-working ventricles have thick, dense walls to support their heavy labor. Gravity pulls as the atria push to send blood down to the ventricles, making their effort considerably easier. The walls of the atria are much thinner. Though the right and left sides of your heart pump your blood to different parts of your body, they beat to the same rhythm. In a normal adult heart, there is no direct connection between the right and left sides of the heart. Blood enters the atria through large veins (the inferior and superior *venae cavae*) and leaves the ventricles through large arteries (the *pulmonary artery* and the *aorta*).

It Pumps You Up

Your heart has just one job: To keep blood flowing through your body's circulatory system—your arteries, veins, and capillaries. It does so through a tightly synchronized series of contractions and relaxations. "Used" blood from the body enters the right atrium through two large veins, the *inferior* and *superior venae cavae*. No, one is not better than the other; the superior *vena cava* brings blood from the upper part of the body, and the inferior *vena cava* brings blood from the lower part of the body. The right atrium contracts to push the blood through the tricuspid valve into the right ventricle, then relaxes. As the blood enters, your heart's electrical system sends the message to squeeze. The ventricle contracts, which causes the valve to the pulmonary artery to open. The contraction forces the blood through the valve, which closes when the right ventricle relaxes. Whew! And all this happens in less than a second!

By Heart
The Latin word *atrium* means "large room" and was what the ancient Romans called the central gathering room of their homes. **Ventricle** comes from the Latin word *ventriculus,* which means "belly." These words are very descriptive—blood enters and fills the atrium, which then releases it to the ventricle. The ventricle propels the blood out into the arteries to carry nourishing oxygen and nutrients to the body.

Take It to Heart
If you're pregnant, you should know that the human heart begins its existence as a narrow tube. By the fourth month of pregnancy, it is fully formed and hard at work. Since the unborn child receives oxygen from its mother via the umbilical cord, the heart bypasses its small, nonfunctioning lungs. Blood flows directly between the two atria through an opening called the *foramen ovale* and between the pulmonary artery and the aorta through an opening called the *ductus arteriosus*. Normally, these openings close at birth when the baby begins breathing. Occasionally they do not, resulting in a congenital heart condition. Often, congenital openings close by themselves over time, though sometimes a surgeon needs to sew them closed.

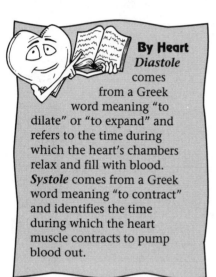

By Heart

Diastole comes from a Greek word meaning "to dilate" or "to expand" and refers to the time during which the heart's chambers relax and fill with blood. *Systole* comes from a Greek word meaning "to contract" and identifies the time during which the heart muscle contracts to pump blood out.

At the same time, the left atrium and ventricle perform a similar dance. The pulmonary veins dump oxygenated blood fresh from the lungs into the left atrium. Contracting at the same time as the right atrium, the left atrium ejects its 2$^1/_2$ or so ounces of blood through the mitral valve into the left ventricle. The left atrium relaxes, the left ventricle contracts (synchronized with its right partner), and the mitral valve closes. The ventricle's contraction forces the blood through the now open aortic valve into the aorta. When the left ventricle relaxes, the aortic valve closes, and the blood pushes out into the arteries and capillaries that take it throughout the body. Doctors call contraction *systole* and relaxation *diastole*.

What Do You Feed a Hungry Heart?

Like other muscles in your body, your heart needs nutrients and exercise. The food you eat feeds your heart as well as the rest of your body. Oxygen nourishes your heart, too. A network of arteries and veins, called *coronary vessels,* covers your heart like vines cover a tree, keeping the heart muscle well-supplied with the nutrients it needs to pump around the clock. Regular, moderate exercise keeps your heart in shape. Strenuous exercise, fear, and sexual activity cause your body to push your heart's "turbo" button, kicking it into high gear. Your heart responds by pumping faster and harder to get more oxygen to the parts of your body that need it, increasing its output as much as fivefold.

Cardiac or vascular (blood vessel) disease (CVD) can fool the heart into thinking it has to work harder all the time. Arteries narrowed by fatty buildup require more pressure to get blood through them. A damaged heart valve that doesn't close all the way leaves some blood behind, so less gets out with each contraction. Your cells notice they're getting a child's portion instead of a full meal and send signals of complaint to your heart. Your heart cranks up its efforts in response and, over time, "bulks up" just like any muscle. Bigger isn't always stronger, however, and an enlarged heart often works less efficiently because the underlying problem still exists. So it works harder, gets bigger, pumps less efficiently... well, you can see where this leads (straight to the cardiologist, do not pass Go, do not collect $200...).

In a Heart Beat

The entire sequence of contraction and relaxation takes your heart about eight-tenths of a second—far less time than it takes you to read about it! This cardiac cycle takes place 70 to 80 times a minute. And while that 2$^1/_2$ ounces of blood your left ventricle sends out with each contraction may seem like a light load, your heart circulates 5 quarts a minute—75 gallons an hour. At that rate, blood leaving your heart reaches your big toe in less time than it takes you to reach down and scratch it.

Heart Sounds: Lubb-Dupp

Though you don't hear it, your heart is a noisy pump. It tells quite a story to your doctor, who can listen in on it with a stethoscope. Your doctor can hear how fast your heart is beating, of course. Comparing that rate with your pulse rate can offer clues about the condition of your arteries. When the valves in your heart open and close, they produce the classic "lubb-dupp" sound—the tricuspid and mitral valves in the atria "lubb," and the aortic and pulmonary valves in the ventricles "dupp." If there's someone nearby who's willing to let you put your ear on his or her chest, you can hear these basic heart sounds (sometimes called the *first* and *second* sounds) yourself.

Sometimes your doctor hears a low-pitched sound after the dupp. If you're under age 30, this is just another sound. If you're over 30, this third sound may signal heart failure. Muscle abnormalities, like those resulting from high blood pressure, produce a fourth low-pitched sound that your doctor hears just before the lubb. Valves that don't close completely make rasping or blowing noises called *murmurs*. Murmurs are common; in the absence of other symptoms, they require no treatment beyond a notation in your medical record. Clicks and snaps reveal other heart conditions, rounding out your heart's repertoire of audible clues about its health.

Red Alert!

If you have a heart murmur, tell your dentist. While a slight murmur may not be noticeable to you, ask your doctor or dentist if you should take antibiotics before dental procedures. Even healthy gums sometimes bleed during cleaning, allowing bacteria normally in the mouth to enter the bloodstream. Persons with heart murmurs have a slightly higher risk of developing an infection around the involved heart valve, which can be a serious medical situation.

Take It to Heart

The sounds a stethoscope detects reveal your heart's secrets to your doctor, aiding diagnosis. This clever instrument is a relatively modern invention, coming about by accident in 1816. French physician René Laënnec rolled a piece of paper into a tube and placed it against the chest of a patient who was too, well, bountiful for him to tap his fingers against the chest to listen for accumulated fluids as was the practice of the day. Within 20 years, the stethoscope was a mainstay of medicine, evolving from a wooden or metal cylinder to today's familiar Y-shaped tubing with earpieces.

Contents Under Pressure

One reason your body's circulatory system functions so efficiently is that it's under pressure. Its pressure levels change as your heart contracts and relaxes. The highest pressure occurs during the systolic phase of the cardiac cycle (contraction). The lower pressure reading occurs during the diastolic phase (relaxation). We measure blood pressure in millimeters of mercury—the number of millimeters that the systolic and diastolic phases cause a column of mercury to rise in the tube of an instrument called a *sphygmomanometer*. Sphygmomanometers also come in models that use mechanical pressure dials and electronic (digital) measuring systems.

By Heart
You may know a *sphygmoma-nometer* by its more familiar term: blood pressure cuff. A sphygmomanometer includes an inflatable cuff that wraps around your upper arm, a bulb attached to a tube to pump the cuff full of air, and a gauge that shows the level of pressure in your arteries as your heart beats.

Measuring your blood pressure is much easier than pronouncing the name of the instrument that does the work. An inflatable cuff goes around your upper arm. When pumped up, it briefly stops the flow of blood through your artery. The doctor or nurse holds a stethoscope over the artery near the surface of the inside of your elbow, just below the cuff, then slowly releases the air in the cuff. The first point at which your pulse can be heard is your systolic pressure, and the last is your diastolic pressure. These numbers appear as one over the other, always systolic over diastolic: 120/70, for example. Normal blood pressure ranges from 90/60 to 140/80. If either number is consistently higher than these ranges, you have high blood pressure. Some people have lower readings that usually require no treatment unless they also have problems at the same time, such as dizziness or fainting.

Untreated high blood pressure can cause stroke, heart failure, and damage to the kidney and *retina* (the back of the eye). High blood pressure is often called the silent killer, because it has no clear symptoms (other than high blood pressure readings). Your risk for high blood pressure goes up if you smoke or are overweight; your risk lowers if you stop smoking and lose weight. Morning headaches and dizziness sometimes indicate high blood pressure, so follow up with your doctor if you have these symptoms. Regular checks are the best way to keep tabs on your blood pressure. We'll talk more about high blood pressure in Chapter 8, "When Your Pressure's Up."

Wired for Life

The heart has its own personal electrical system that triggers it to contract. While this system doesn't generate enough juice to light a lamp, it does spark a series of contractions that sends your blood on its journey through your body. These tiny jolts of electricity originate in the *sinoatrial node*, a pea-sized cluster of special-duty cells at the right atrium, and ripple through your heart muscle to initiate each cardiac cycle. A smaller second node, the *atrioventricular*, serves as a relay station and emergency backup if the sinoatrial node stops working. Your doctor can create a picture of the electrical patterns of your heart with an *electrocardiogram* (EKG, sometimes ECG; more on this in Chapter 6, "Straight to the Heart"). Electrodes attached to your chest transmit your heart's electrical activity to a machine that produces a graph-like recording. An EKG is painless and takes only a few minutes. Heart rhythm problems can make your heart beat too fast (*tachycardia*) or too slow (*bradycardia*).Heart block, a common form of heart disease, occurs when something interferes with the heart's electrical system. This interference knocks the synchronization between the atria and the ventricles out of whack. Mild heart block may cause no symptoms and require no treatment. In moderate or severe heart block, the atria and ventricles beat at different rhythms. A telltale slow, steady pulse that stays at the same rate even with exercise provides evidence of medically significant heart block. Other symptoms may include dizziness and fainting. Doctors use pacemakers and medications to treat heart rhythm problems.

Red Alert!

You're at greatest risk of sudden cardiac death from disruption of your heart's electrical system in the first few minutes to hours after a heart attack occurs. Get to a hospital emergency room immediately if you experience symptoms of a heart attack!

It's in Your Blood

Your blood may look like a homogenous red fluid, but it's much more. Four distinct components combine to make blood:

➤ **Red blood cells** or *erythrocytes*, which get their color from the hemoglobin they carry, give blood its red color.

➤ **White blood cells** or *leukocytes* are the body's infection-fighting warriors.

➤ **Platelets**, colorless, sticky knights, race to the rescue whenever you cut yourself.

➤ **Plasma**, a straw-colored fluid, transports the other components and keeps the blood vessels from collapsing.

Take It to Heart

What's your blood type? While all blood looks the same, the microscope reveals important differences in the molecules on the surface of red blood cells, which are identified as A or B. Red blood cells that have only A molecules are type A; those with only B molecules are type B. Those with both molecules are type AB, and those with neither are type O. Your blood type becomes important if you need a blood transfusion, because the blood you receive must be compatible with your type.

Take It to Heart

Are you positive or negative? This matters, too. If your blood has a certain protein, it's called *Rh positive*. If it doesn't, it's Rh negative. The Rh stands for *rhesus*, the monkey species in which the protein was first discovered. Positive and negative don't mix. Sometimes an unborn baby can inherit Rh-positive blood from its father while its mother is Rh negative, in which case the mother's blood produces antigens that can attack the baby's blood. If an Rh-negative mother has an Rh-positive baby, doctors give the mother antibodies at the time of the birth, to prevent problems in future pregnancies.

Somewhat doughnut-shaped, red blood cells are the pack mules of your blood. The hemoglobin they contain functions like a chemical saddle, carrying oxygen and other nutrients to body tissues and carbon dioxide, the waste product of cell activity, away to the lungs for disposal. A milliliter of blood, an amount the thickness and diameter of a dime, contains about 5 million red blood cells. Though the average red blood cell lives only 120 days, it makes nearly 350,000 trips through the heart during its lifetime. Even when it dies, the red blood cell contributes to life; the body reuses most of its molecules as nutrients for other cell activities. Your body continuously makes new red blood cells. The "recipe" your bone marrow uses to do this includes iron, amino acids, folic acid, and vitamin B12.

Cardio Care

A recent study suggests that donating blood may decrease your chances of certain kinds of heart disease by controlling the level of platelets, responsible for clotting, in your blood. Healthy adults can donate blood every two months without risk. Your body replaces the lost fluid volume within hours and the lost cells within days.

White blood cells, also called *white corpuscles* or *leukocytes*, are the warriors of your blood. They rush to surround and devour bacteria, viruses, and other threats that can enter the bloodstream. There are far fewer white than red blood cells—only about 7,500 per milliliter. Your blood's knights in sticky armor are the platelets, which swarm to the location of any cut to plug the flow of blood. The resulting clump is called a *clot*, which hardens into a scab as exposure to air dries it. Clots can also form inside a blood vessel, often as the result of a bruise or other injury. If it is big enough, such a clot can block blood from flowing through the vessel. Tissues on the other side of the clot no longer receive life-giving oxygen, and they die. When this happens in the brain, it's called a stroke. Stroke can have serious consequences, including paralysis, speech impairment, and even death. We'll talk more about stroke in Chapter 9, "Stroke: Brain Attack."

Plasma is to your blood what a stream is to fish. This straw-colored liquid rushes your blood's various components (cells, nutrients, salts, proteins) to their destinations. Plasma is 95 percent water, and it also provides the volume your blood vessels need to keep them from collapsing. Remember those eight or so glasses of water you're supposed to drink every day? That's not just to test your bladder capacity. Your body replenishes plasma continuously from the fluids you drink. It's so efficient that when you donate blood, your body replaces the lost fluid volume with fresh plasma by the time you leave the donor center.

Go with the Flow

Arteries, veins, and capillaries form the highway system that speeds blood through your body. Connected together, they'd cover 100,000 miles—the equivalent of more than a dozen trips between Los Angeles and Boston! Some are quite large, like the *aorta* (the artery leading away from your heart), which can measure more than an inch across. Others are hard to see even with a microscope, so fine that blood cells must squeeze through single file. Arteries and veins run parallel to each other, often shadowing bones for protection. Capillaries stretch like a web through body tissues to connect arteries and veins, making your circulatory system a closed network.

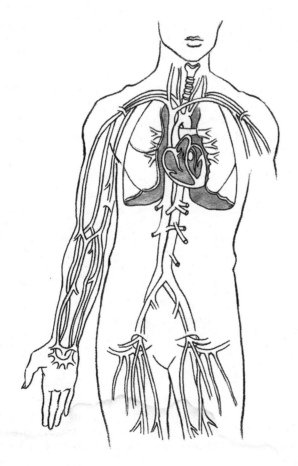

The arteries, veins, and capillaries that make up your body's circulatory system maintain a constant flow of blood throughout your body.

Arteries carry oxygen-rich blood from the heart to your body's organs and systems. Their muscular walls expand to accept the blood the heart forces into them when it contracts. When the heart relaxes, the pressure in the arteries keeps the blood moving forward. The blood moves through the body quite rapidly and efficiently; remember, it takes less than half a minute for blood to make it all the way through your circulatory system and back to the heart.

Most arteries are deep inside the body, snuggled into dense muscle tissue or hugging bones to shelter them from outside dangers like cuts and punctures. A wound that opens an artery is very serious, since it can drain large amounts of blood in just minutes. At certain places in your body, the arteries are closer to the surface—like the inside of your wrist, your neck at the base of your jaw, and your groin. Press on one of these points, and you can feel your pulse, the rhythm of the artery's contraction and expansion. Because your arteries beat in harmony with your heart, your pulse provides quick clues about what's going on with your heart.

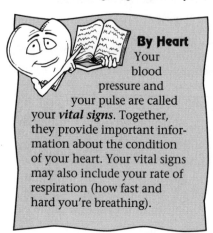

By Heart
Your blood pressure and your pulse are called your *vital signs*. Together, they provide important information about the condition of your heart. Your vital signs may also include your rate of respiration (how fast and hard you're breathing).

Veins bring back the waste (like carbon dioxide) that your body's cells generate as they go about the activities that keep your body healthy and functioning. The easiest way for your body to get blood back to your heart would be to have you stand on your head 70 times a minute or so to let gravity do its thing. Since this would mess up your hair and make you quite dizzy, your body's architecture provides an ingenious solution: valves. One-way valves inside your veins keep your blood from following the pull of gravity and keep it moving toward your heart. Your veins also get helpful squeezes from your muscles.

Capillaries extend deep into body tissues, linking your arteries and veins. Blood cells pass nutrients to and collect waste from other cells through the very thin capillary walls. When you get a small cut on your finger, the blood that oozes out comes from the capillaries. Because they are so tiny, capillaries were the last piece of the circulation puzzle that medical scientists discovered.

The Beat Goes On

It doesn't take much to make a big difference to your heart health... though those little things you let slip (like the walk you'll take tomorrow) can eventually add up to big problems. Though a heart attack may strike suddenly, the events preparing your heart to rebel take a long time to develop. Treat your heart well, and it'll stay happy and healthy for many years. And there's no time like now to start. A recent study indicates that people who take a brisk, 30-minute walk at least six times a month can add years to their lives. Less than twice a week is a pretty small investment for such a big gain! You do even more for your heart—and your sense of well-being—if you get 30 minutes of moderate exercise four or five days a week.

Much of what your heart needs to stay healthy is good for you all over. And what's good for you all over is good for your heart. Exercise, massage, drinking plenty of water, getting enough rest—these things all improve your general health and well-being, and that makes your heart happy. You don't have to be a world-class athlete to have a body that's fit and a heart that's strong. As you'll see in upcoming chapters, heart-healthy living is a matter of choice and balance.

The Least You Need to Know

- ➤ Your heart is a powerful, efficient pump that keeps your body alive and well.
- ➤ Blood is the mother lode of life, rich in nutrients your cells need to carry on the work of living. An extensive network of arteries, veins, and capillaries transports blood throughout your body.
- ➤ A few simple procedures—feeling your pulse, measuring your blood pressure, and listening to the sounds of your heart—give your doctor a wealth of information about the condition of your heart.
- ➤ Regular exercise (even just walking) significantly lowers your pulse and blood pressure, allowing your heart to live a longer, happier life.

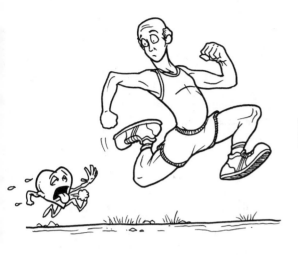

Keeping Pace

Once upon a time, not so long ago, really, few people died of heart disease. Before the 1900s, days started and ended with physical activity. Most jobs involved some form of manual labor, if only carrying boxes of papers from an office to a storeroom. The only wheels were on trains and bicycles; no matter where you were going, you got there by walking. Housework was truly hard work—scrubbing laundry on a washboard, beating rugs, and splitting firewood were but a few of the typical everyday chores. Then came the Industrial Age, and everything changed. Machines took over tasks like laundry and heating the house. Cars took over for feet, elevators replaced stairs, and automation reduced manual labor. And heart disease moved into first place as the cause of death among adult Americans.

Do You Live in Your Heart or in Your Head?

Without question, technology has given us many significant improvements. Diseases like smallpox and polio, which once claimed thousands of lives every year, now are such rarities (thanks to vaccines to prevent them) that new doctors may have never seen a case

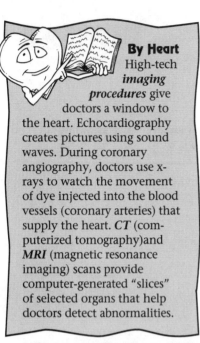

By Heart
High-tech *imaging procedures* give doctors a window to the heart. Echocardiography creates pictures using sound waves. During coronary angiography, doctors use x-rays to watch the movement of dye injected into the blood vessels (coronary arteries) that supply the heart. *CT* (computerized tomography) and *MRI* (magnetic resonance imaging) scans provide computer-generated "slices" of selected organs that help doctors detect abnormalities.

of either. The mysteries of the working heart that fascinated yet eluded Hippocrates, Galen, and William Harvey are no more, revealed by open heart surgery and amazing imaging procedures that let doctors "see" the heart at work. Modern medicine, it seems, can mend just about anything. It's this mindset, say those who study health trends, that leads us to believe we can eat, drink, and make merry to our heart's desire because the doctor will fix us when we break.

What your heart really desires, of course, is for you to take care of it to the best of your ability—not to rely on your doctor to put you back together again. It's easy to live in your brain, with its reassuring messages that no matter what you do, there's always tomorrow. To keep those tomorrows coming, however, you need to move your lifestyle to a "better" neighborhood—your heart. And your heart doesn't ask that much of you, really. Just that you nourish it, exercise it, and shelter it from stress—all the things the rest of you wants, too!

Life in the Fast Lane

If leisure means nothing more to you than a funky suit from the days of disco dancing, you're not alone. Studies show that the 9-to-5 workday is a myth for most Americans. Shift work, take-home work, and extended hours are more the norm than the exception in today's work environment. Over the last 20 years, the average workweek has lengthened by more than three hours, draining nearly 160 hours a year from other activities. Family responsibilities have their daily demands, too, from fixing dinner and chores to helping the kids with homework. Oddly, we strive to get ourselves into this fast lane, thinking that's where we'll find our share of the good life. Problem is, life isn't all that good when there's no time left to enjoy it. The race to keep up with the fast pace of modern living takes its toll on our bodies, from reducing the amount of sleep we get each night to raising blood pressure and pulse rates.

Finding Center

Is stress the essence of your lifestyle? Continuous stress keeps your body in a "fight or flight" mode, with your brain constantly signaling your adrenal glands to sound the warning to your heart: "Crank it up so we can get out of here!" Like the unfortunate boy who cried wolf one too many times, your heart eventually wearies of the alarms and responds by staying in a state of acceleration. The resulting higher pulse and blood pressure fool your brain for a while, then the cycle starts again. Eventually, your heart works so hard to get blood to other organ systems that it short-changes itself.

The resulting condition is called *myocardial ischemia*, and it can have no symptoms yet permanently damage muscle tissue in your heart.

One way to break this "fight or flight" cycle is to take 10 minutes or so several times a day to think about what's going on with your body. This is called *centering*, and even if you do nothing else, it will calm you. Take 10 now and give it a try. You don't have to do anything special, just sit quietly (you can close your eyes as long as you promise to stay awake) and think about how your body feels. Of course, we encourage you to engage in other activities to improve your heart's long-term health, too.

Keep Moving!

How active is active enough? Put a check beside the items you think are necessary for heart-healthy exercise:

- ❏ Fashionable running clothes and expensive shoes to match
- ❏ An electronic home fitness gym, complete with stair-stepper and fingertip pulse oximeter
- ❏ Lessons in the hottest aerobic dance moves
- ❏ A personal trainer and complete fitness program
- ❏ 28 hours in every day

Of course, it would be nice to have all these things, especially those extra four hours a day. But don't wait for them to start exercising, because you don't need them. If channel surfing wears you out, you live what doctors call a *sedentary lifestyle*—and you have lots of company. More than 40 percent of Americans get so little exercise in their daily lives that walking up a flight of stairs leaves them winded. The biggest excuse we offer for not exercising? C'mon, all together now: "I haven't got time." You may feel that your life is already moving so fast you can barely keep up. Believe it or not, getting your body moving makes it easier! The truth is, it doesn't take much time or extra effort to add activity to your life. And if you're part of the 20 percent of Americans who get enough exercise, give yourself a pat on the back and keep on moving.

Cardio Care
Studies show that walking for just six 30-minute periods a month can add years to your life. Even short walks of 10 minutes or so throughout the day add up to big benefits for your heart and your health.

Does life in the fast lane have your time gridlocked? The easiest activity you can do is something you do, at least to some extent, every day anyway. Walk. But don't just walk from the couch to the refrigerator or from your car to the parking-garage elevator. Put some zip in your steps! A brisk walk is good for the heart and the mind. Here are three quick ways to squeeze walking into your busy schedule:

➤ Take the stairs instead of the elevator, up and down.

➤ Park a block or two away from work, or at the back of the parking lot at the grocery store.

➤ Visit co-workers in your office instead of sending e-mail or voice mail messages.

Do you like to dance? Then by all means, shake, shimmy, scoot, or swing! Enjoy gardening and yard work? These activities can help keep your body in shape, too. Even common chores like washing floors and vacuuming can get your heart pounding and your blood flowing. So whatever else you do, keep moving! Your heart's health and happiness depend on it.

Your Finger on the Pulse

In Edgar Allan Poe's classic short story, "The Tell-Tale Heart," a murderer begins to hear his victim's heartbeat as the police come to search the house where the victim lies buried beneath the floor. The throbbing grows louder and louder, until the murderer can hear nothing else and shouts his confession to the startled police officers, who had heard nothing and had been about to leave.

In reality, your pulse is a tattletale of sorts, blabbing your heart's secrets to those who can "hear" them by feeling your pulse rate. When you're calm and resting, your pulse maintains a comfortable cadence of 70 to 100 beats per minute, steady and regular. When you're exercising or stressed, your pulse climbs and can become less consistent. Sudden fear can make you feel like you've stepped into *The Tell-Tale Heart* as the pounding of your heart fills your ears—though what you actually hear is the blood rushing through the major arteries in your upper neck. And it's common (and normal) to hear your heartbeat when you're calm and quiet, like right before you fall asleep. Generally, your blood pressure rises when your pulse rate does, though the reverse is not necessarily the case.

How to Measure Your Heart Rate

All you need to take your pulse is a watch with a second hand and two fingers (not your thumb, which has a perceptible pulse of its own that will confuse your count). And of course, an artery near the surface of your body so you can feel it. Two that work well are the carotid artery in your neck just below your jawbone and the radial artery on the thumb side of the inside of your wrist. Your pulse is the number of times your heart beats in a minute. You can count the beats for a full minute, or count the beats for 30 seconds and multiply by two.

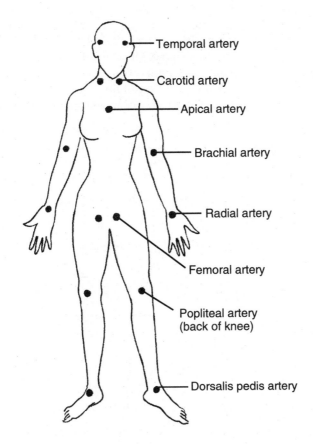

Temporal artery

Carotid artery

Apical artery

Brachial artery

Radial artery

Femoral artery

Popliteal artery
(back of knee)

Dorsalis pedis artery

*You can feel your
pulse at places
where an artery is
near the surface of
your body.*

To take your pulse at your wrist, follow these steps:

1. Sit down. Put your left arm on a table or other surface, palm up. Relax. Place your clock or watch with a second hand where you can see it easily.

2. Press down with your index and middle fingers on the inside of your wrist on the thumb side, just below the base of your thumb. Do you feel your pulse? If not, move your fingers slightly up or down your wrist until you do.

3. Practice feeling your pulse under your fingertips, and count a few beats to get a sense of your pulse's rhythm.

4. Watch the second hand on your clock or watch. When it gets to the 12 or the 6 (make it easy for yourself!), start counting the beats for real. Count for a full minute.

5. Record your resting heart rate: _____ beats per minute.

The resting heart rate for most adults is between 60 and 100 beats per minute. Athletes whose bodies are exceptionally well-conditioned may have a resting heart rate lower than 60. If you take your pulse while your arm is elevated above your heart (while you are standing, for example), you might get a false result.

An athlete often uses the carotid artery to measure resting and target pulse rates, since it provides an accurate rate in virtually any position. The carotid artery is also much larger than the radial artery and is easier to find in a hurry. The carotid is the artery medics reach for as a quick determination of a patient's status. You can easily feel the pulse in your femoral artery in your groin, too, though you're certain to get some odd looks and probably a few less-than-kind comments if you reach inside your pants to check your pulse.

Feeling your pulse at the carotid, femoral, and radial arteries.

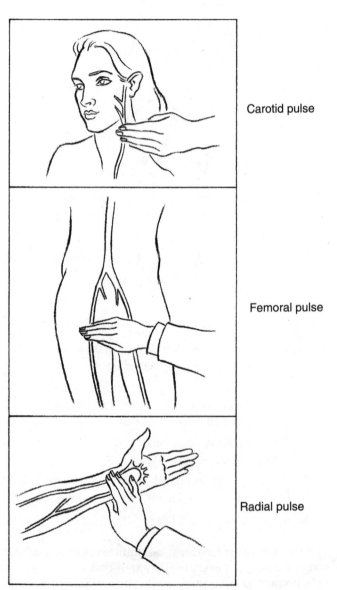

Carotid pulse

Femoral pulse

Radial pulse

What Makes Your Heart Race?

Many factors affect your pulse, from physical activity to anxiety or nervousness. Your resting pulse rate tells how regularly and consistently your heart pumps when your body is doing little more than simply living. Your heart reacts to signals your body sends when your tissues need more oxygen and nutrients, pumping faster and harder to meet your body's demands. It's normal for your pulse rate to slow when you're at rest and to increase when you exercise or when you're feeling stressed.

Sometimes you might feel that your heart is pounding or fluttering. Caffeine (in soft drinks, coffee, and tea), nicotine (in cigarettes and other tobacco products), and stress are common causes of this sensation, called a *palpitation*. Though your heart feels like it stops for a moment and then takes off again, it's really just experiencing variations in rhythm called *ectopic* heart beats. Palpitations can have several causes, including.

➤ **Drugs:** Caffeine (in soft drinks, coffee, and tea) and nicotine (in cigarettes and other tobacco products).

➤ **Stress.**

➤ **Hyperthyroidism** (an overactive thyroid gland): One of several medical conditions that can cause your heart to beat faster than normal.

➤ **Arrythmias:** Rhythm abnormalities caused by electrical irregularities in the heart.

➤ **Atrial tachycardia:** A common arrhythmia where the heart's upper chambers or atria suddenly accelerate.

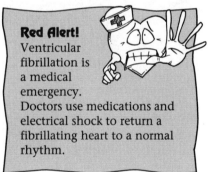

By Heart
Bradycardia (Latin for "slow heart") describes a heart rate that is slower than normal. *Tachycardia* (Latin for "fast heart") describes a heart rate that is faster than normal. *Fibrillation* is a very rapid, disorganized beating. When a ventricle fibrillates, as sometimes happens following a heart attack, the heart cannot pump effectively.

Red Alert!
Ventricular fibrillation is a medical emergency. Doctors use medications and electrical shock to return a fibrillating heart to a normal rhythm.

Your doctor should evaluate palpitations that last for more than a few minutes, happen several times over a day or so, leave you feeling faint or like you can't catch your breath, or cause chest pain.

How do you know if your heart is working too hard when you exercise? Two simple tests can tell you whether you're exercising too vigorously or too lightly:

➤ **Talk test:** Can you walk (or exercise) and talk at the same time? If not, you're pushing your heart too hard.

Just for YOU
Do you have anxiety or panic attacks? About 6 percent of the American population does, and palpitations are one of the most common symptoms that cause people to see a doctor. While panic attacks are frightening, they aren't dangerous for your heart. Your doctor will take a careful history and maybe run a few tests to be sure your palpitations are related to anxiety or panic attacks. Treatment may include medication for the anxiety and counseling for related emotional issues.

By Heart
Your *resting pulse rate* tells how fast and hard your heart beats when you're not doing anything strenuous. For most adults, this is between 60 and 100. Your *maximum heart rate* is the fastest and hardest your heart can pump without going into fibrillation, and differs according to age. Your *target heart rate* is the pulse you need to maintain to give your heart a good workout. It is 50 to 75 percent of your maximum heart rate.

➤ **Singing test:** Can you walk and sing? What matters is not whether you can carry a tune but whether you can carry out the process of singing, which requires good effort from your lungs. If so, step up your pace a bit to give your heart a decent workout.

A more precise measure of how hard your heart is working is your target heart rate or pulse, which is 50 to 75 percent of your maximum heart rate. Maximum and target heart rates vary according to your age. In general, you can ballpark your maximum heart rate by subtracting your age from 220. For example, if you're 45 years old, your maximum heart rate is approximately 175 beats per minute, and your target heart rate is 88 to 131 beats per minute. When your activity is strenuous enough to put your pulse at your target heart rate, your cardiovascular system (heart, lungs, and circulation) is getting a good workout. It takes time and conditioning to feel comfortable exercising at your target heart rate, so let your body work up to it.

Calculating Your Target Heart Rate

1. 220 – Your Age: _____ = Your Maximum Heart Rate: _____

2. Your Target Heart Rate: _____ × .5 = _____

3. Your Target Heart Rate: _____ × .75 = _____

4. Your Target Heart Rate = _____ to _____ beats per minute (the range between your calculations in step 2 and step 3).

Homeostasis: Achieving a Healthy Balance

Your body systems strive to maintain a constant environment for themselves regardless of what's going on outside your body. Doctors call this process of self-adjustment *homeostasis*. Some body functions that stay in this state of equilibrium are blood sugar levels, body temperature, and blood pressure. Body systems achieve homeostasis automatically, making adjustments to compensate for changes. Your heart rate increases when your blood pressure falls, pumping blood faster to bring your blood pressure back up. Low oxygen levels in your blood signal your lungs and heart to increase their efforts. Some disease conditions interfere with homeostasis. In the presence of diabetes, the body can no longer regulate blood sugar levels. In hypertension, blood pressure is too high, and the body's mechanisms that control it no longer work to bring it down. In some situations, conscious actions on your part can assist homeostasis. Exercise, diet, and weight loss can reduce high blood pressure and lower your heart rate so your heart doesn't have to work so hard.

Sometimes we develop unhealthy patterns that feel balanced but really aren't. You might feel comfortable starting your morning with a double tall latté because it doesn't have a noticeable effect (unless you don't have it...). It's not that the caffeine is somehow good for your body. Your body has simply developed a tolerance for (some say a dependence on) this daily dose of stimulant. Doing the right things—eating right, exercising regularly—to achieve a healthy homeostasis can take a period of mental and physical adjustment while your body makes the shift from juggling your bad habits to balancing your healthy ones.

Body, mind, and spirit strive for homeostasis as well. We yearn for balance in a world that sorely lacks it. Some people reach for this balance from the mind and spirit through meditation and prayer. Others start with the body, using running, bicycling, dance, and other strenuous activities to become "at one" with themselves. Those who've already figured out the connection pursue disciplines like yoga and the martial arts that link the mind and the body through movements that exercise both. No matter where you start, the ultimate goal is the same: to transcend the stresses of everyday life and achieve a sense of physical, mental, and spiritual tranquillity. We know this balance—homeostasis—as health.

> **Red Alert!**
> Some medical conditions lower the maximum heart rate, as do certain medications (particularly some used to treat high blood pressure). If you have a medical condition or take regular medication, get the go-ahead from your doctor before you start an exercise program.

> **By Heart**
> The words *medicine* and *meditate* come from the same original Latin root, *mede,* which means "take appropriate measures." From this root, the Latin word for "to think about" became *meditari,* and the word for "look after, heal" became *medere.*

What Does Breathing Have to Do with It?

Breathing is obviously a vital activity. Without it, the oxygen–carbon dioxide exchange that sustains life cannot take place. Breathing brings oxygen from the air into your lungs, where your red blood cells turn over carbon dioxide in trade. A man's lungs hold about $1^{1}/_{2}$ gallons of air at a time, while a woman's smaller lungs hold about 1 gallon. Normal breathing (at rest) brings just under a pint of fresh air into the lungs, while a good deep breath brings in up to eight times as much. The air you breathe is not all oxygen; in fact, it's not even mostly oxygen. Air is typically 78 percent nitrogen, 21 percent oxygen, and the rest a blend of other gases and water vapor. The average adult takes 12 to 18 breaths a minute at rest and can breathe up to 80 times a minute during strenuous exercise.

The Heart-Lung Connection

The heart-lung connection is essential for life. Without it, or when it's disrupted, cells fail to receive the oxygen they need to function, and they die. That's not so good for you, either! A good relationship between your heart and your lungs is essential for your well-being. Your heart may send your blood pulsing through your blood vessels, but this won't do much good without the lungs to exchange carbon dioxide for oxygen.

Take It to Heart

The ancient Greek physician Galen believed the arteries carried not blood but *pneuma*, or air. So did Western physicians who followed him, until many centuries later, when Michael Servetus (1511–53) offered the then heretical notion that the heart sent blood to the lungs, which filled the blood with oxygen and returned it to the heart. This departure from contemporary thinking about the circulatory system earned Servetus the wrath of his contemporaries. Despite the unpopularity of his assertion in his time, Servetus was, as we know today, correct.

Just for YOU

Teens and young adults seldom think of themselves as candidates for heart disease. Yet research shows that the disease process begins at this age or earlier. Young people tend to be less physically active, particularly if they're no longer in school; eat more high-fat junk food; and smoke more than their mortality-conscious elders—all behaviors that increase the likelihood of heart disease.

Smoking is one of the most damaging things you can do to your lungs. As your heart sees it, smoking is a particularly devastating habit because it decreases the lungs' ability to exchange carbon monoxide (CO) and oxygen. Smoking produces carbon monoxide, which swirls into the lungs with every drag from a cigarette. Carbon monoxide binds more easily with the hemoglobin in red blood cells, effectively "bumping" oxygen molecules aside. Your cells can't use carbon monoxide, so its presence keeps the red blood cells from transporting cell waste (carbon dioxide) to the lungs as well. The tar residue tobacco smoke leaves behind clogs the tiny sacs, or *alveoli*, where the oxygen–carbon dioxide exchange takes place. Your lungs have about 600 million of these minuscule exchange centers, which look like clusters of balloons under a microscope. Don't delude yourself into thinking that with so many, plugging a few thousand or even million won't matter. It does, reducing the efficiency of your lungs in ways that you feel as shortness of breath. The good news about smoking is that once you quit, many of the damaged alveoli recover. We'll talk more about smoking in Chapters 4, "The Heart Knows No Boundaries," and 21, "Light Up Your Heart, Not a Cigarette."

Take a Deep Breath

Go ahead, take a deep breath, right now. No one will notice—breathing is normal, and deep breathing is common in these stressful times. Take your time with this deep breath, though. Breathe in… hold it… breathe out. Surprised to feel a little more relaxed, a little more alert, a little less stressed? Go ahead, take another if you like. Here's the most amazing part: There's not much else you can do that gives you so much benefit for so little effort! Breathing revitalizes your body and soothes your anxious mind.

Breathing techniques have been used in many cultures for many purposes. Athletes use breathing to help them reach peak performance. Childbirth classes incorporate patterns of breathing to help women cope with the pain of labor and delivery and focus on the birthing process. Breathing is central to various Eastern philosophical systems like Taoism, in which practitioners spend years mastering techniques that emphasize breathing from the soles of the feet—using the whole body, not just the nose and chest, to breathe. But no matter what your level of physical or spiritual fitness, breathing techniques improve your health by lowering your stress levels.

Opening the Mind-Body Connection

What if we told you that you hold the key to a happy, healthy heart… not in the palm of your hand, but in your mind? Obviously, heart disease is no figment of your imagination, and wishing won't make it go away. But there's a phenomenal connection between your mind and your body. Your mind can influence, even change, much of what happens in and to your body—if you let it. What doctors once scorned as hocus-pocus now has scientific validity. Methods like biofeedback and self-hypnosis produce measurable changes in physical functions such as pulse and blood pressure. Neuroscientist David Felten discovered that there are nerve threads that connect the nervous and immune systems in the body, much as capillaries connect arteries and veins. This discovery could explain why a nasty cold or other physical ailments often follows a bad case of the blues. And scientists have long known about mood-altering chemical substances found naturally in the body, such as endorphins and neuropeptides. Perhaps an ancient Chinese proverb says it best: "When the mind is present in the heart, we call it happiness."

By Heart
Endorphins are natural substances, chemically similar to morphine, that your brain releases to relieve pain. Endorphins are responsible for the sense of euphoria known as "runner's high." *Neuropeptides* are stings of amino acids that carry molecular messages from your brain to your cells.

The Least You Need to Know

➤ Heart disease is a phenomenon of modern times.

➤ Move, move, move! A body in motion has a healthier, happier heart.

➤ You can easily calculate your resting, target, and maximum heart rates.

➤ Stress hurts your heart. Just one deep breath sends oxygen to your blood, slows your heart rate, and centers you.

➤ There is a powerful—and healing—connection between your mind and your body.

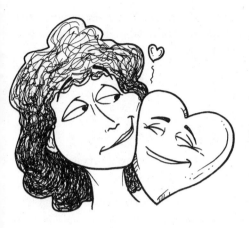

The Heart Knows No Boundaries

How many warning lights are lit on the dashboard of your car? How about that little gas pump inside your fuel gauge? That's an easy one to ignore—after all, you know how far your car can go on fumes. What about that yellow light, reminding you that it's time for an oil change? The oil's a bit dirty, sure, and the level's at the bottom "OK" line on the dipstick. You'll get it changed next week, when things slow down at work and your kids no longer need your chauffeur services. After all, the light's not red yet, so you have some time. Those red lights usually get our attention, though, especially that one that means "pull over and stop NOW or this car will self-destruct."

It's not so important that you know what your car's warning lights mean as it is that you know they signal a problem that needs your attention. Now. Not on the way home, or tomorrow, or next week when life is less hectic. The same is true of the warning "lights" your heart sends you. Do you feel winded after climbing a flight of stairs? This could be a yellow warning from your heart that it doesn't have the fuel (oxygen and nutrients) to meet the extra demands of your adventure in physical activity. Has your doctor told you your blood pressure's a little high, yet you still can't find time to get in some exercise?

This yellow warning soon will turn red unless you make the time. Do you experience pain in your chest after strenuous exercise? This couldn't be more of a red alert if it sent off bells and alarms. You may well have moderate to serious heart disease, putting you at risk for catastrophic "self-destruct" if you fail to respond immediately. (Remember, chest pain or discomfort that lasts more than a few minutes can signal a heart attack. Don't ignore this warning—get medical attention immediately.)

What Happens If You Ignore Your Heart?

How do you respond when that ominous "all systems failure" warning lights up on your dash? (Be honest—we won't tell anyone!)

A. I immediately pull to the side of the road, stop the car, and turn off the engine, like the owner's manual says, and use my cell phone to call for help.

B. I make my way over to the slow lane while searching my glove box for the owner's manual (I know it's in there somewhere) to see what I'm supposed to do.

C. Geez, I can't pull over right now! I'm late for work, and I have that big presentation, and besides, nothing happened last week when the light flashed on and off. I just kept driving, and everything was fine.

D. Warning light? What warning light?

Most of us know, of course, that the correct response is A. Given our fill-the-day lifestyles, we're more likely to choose B or C. We're willing to take the risk that the car will get us where we need to go for now. If you selected D, be sure your auto insurance covers towing! Yet the consequences of B, C, or D are likely to be significant. Sure, your car may make it through its current crisis and maybe a few more. Perhaps it has been flashing that light at you for long enough that it seems more like an annoying quirk than a warning. But a problem like a leaking valve can trigger your car's warning system long before you notice the oil loss, long before the engine freezes and the block cracks. Repair the problem now, and you get a bill for a few hundred dollars. Delay, and you'll be replacing an engine to the tune of several thousand dollars—or maybe even your whole car. Ignoring the warning signals your car sends hurts your checkbook. Ignoring the warning signals your heart sends can cost you your lifestyle… or your life.

Who's at Risk for Heart Problems?

Heart problems can happen to anyone, and you're no exception. It doesn't matter whether you're a man or a woman, old or young, living on a farm in Kansas or an apartment in New York City. There are certain circumstances, which doctors call *risk factors*, that make it more or less likely that you'll have heart problems. Doctors divide risks for heart problems into two categories: those you can change and those you can't.

Risks You Can Change

Would it surprise you to learn that six of the most significant risk factors for heart disease are ones you can control? Each of these is so important it has its own chapter, though we'll list them briefly here so you know what they are:

➤ Smoking

➤ High cholesterol

➤ High blood pressure

➤ Physical inactivity

➤ Overweight

➤ Stress

More than 350,000 people die each year from heart disease caused by cigarette smoking, and we don't want you to be one of them. We just have to take a soapbox moment here to say that smoking is one of those activities from which no good comes. Smoking's detrimental effects on health are well documented; there are no known health benefits.

The benefits of quitting start within minutes of your last cigarette and continue for the rest of your life:

➤ In 20 minutes, circulation returns to the blood vessels in your hands and feet as the constricting effect of nicotine wears off.

➤ In 8 hours, your blood's oxygen and carbon monoxide levels are back to normal.

➤ Within a year, the extra risk of heart disease you had as a smoker is half what it was when you smoked.

➤ Within 10 years, your risk of heart disease is no greater than someone who never smoked.

If you don't smoke now or have given it up, great! If you smoke now, stop. (OK, moment's over.)

Controllable risks are so crucial in preventing heart disease not just because you can reduce them by changing your behaviors, though that would certainly be enough by itself. Controllable risks also compound each other. Smoking, lack of exercise, and obesity all affect cholesterol levels. Physical inactivity is a key

Just for YOU
Do you have Type 2 (adult-onset) diabetes? You probably already know how important it is to watch your diet and exercise regularly. Did you know it's also important to watch your heart health? Over 30 percent of adults with Type 2 diabetes already have heart disease by the time their diabetes is diagnosed. Type 2 diabetes is often resistant to insulin, which increases the build-up of plaque in the arteries. If you have diabetes, have your blood pressure checked every three to six months and your blood cholesterol level tested yearly.

element of obesity; add stress to the mix, and you have a recipe for high blood pressure (and Type 2 diabetes, another heart disease risk factor, especially if you're over the age of 50).

There's good news wrapped in this compounding package, too. Once you start working on one risk factor, you chip away at others at the same time. Exercise speeds metabolism, resulting in weight loss and lower cholesterol levels (in combination with improved eating habits). Exercise also reduces stress, which lowers blood pressure.

Risks You're Stuck With

Some risk factors you just can't change. Your age (and the fact that it's increasing). Your gender (sorry, guys). Your family history. Diabetes, if you have it. Heart problems you already have. Men still get the short end of the statistic when it comes to heart problems, until about age 65 or so when women's risk catches up. Decreasing estrogen levels play an important role, partly because estrogen helps keep your cholesterol down. One benefit of post-menopausal estrogen replacement therapy, in fact, is that it somewhat restores this natural protection against heart disease.

If you have any of these risks (and eventually, we all have at least one: aging), don't panic. Knowledge is power, and you know it's especially important for you to control the risk factors you can. A heart-healthy lifestyle gives you the best odds possible for beating heart disease.

What's Your Risk Level? A Self-Quiz

Which risk factors should concern you? Take this quick quiz for a snapshot of your personal heart disease risk level. Choose the answer that most closely describes you:

1. I smoke cigarettes:
   A. Never.
   B. Less than a pack a day.
   C. Two packs or more a day.
   D. I light my next from the one in my mouth.

2. For exercise, I:
   A. Walk, jog, bicycle, swim, or do aerobic dance 30 to 45 minutes, 3 or 4 times a week.
   B. Bicycle or walk to work 3 or 4 times a week.
   C. Sometimes walk the dog after dinner.
   D. Run from the couch to the kitchen during TV commercials.

3. In my family:

   A. The only heart disease is in a great aunt on my mother's side.

   B. My father and two of his brothers have high blood pressure.

   C. My father had a heart attack when I was in high school, his father died of a heart attack before I was born, and his mother died of a stroke when she was 62.

   D. My parents died of heart disease and I, my two sisters, and one brother have high blood pressure.

4. My favorite meal is:

   A. Grilled halibut, homemade rice pilaf, and steamed broccoli, with angel food cake and strawberries for dessert.

   B. Vegetarian lasagna and a green salad with raspberry vinaigrette dressing, with peach cobbler and low-fat ice cream for dessert.

   C. Pizza and beer.

   D. Prime rib, baked potato with the works, mushrooms sautéed in butter and wine, a little of everything from the salad bar, and chocolate decadence cake for dessert.

5. When I finish an especially challenging project, I reward myself with:

   A. A swim at the pool, a bicycle ride, in-line skating, a game of basketball, an extra round of golf, or Frisbee fetch with my dog.

   B. The afternoon off and a massage.

   C. Nothing—it's on to the next one.

   D. A bucket of fried chicken, a beer, and control of the TV remote.

6. My age is:

   A. Under 30.

   B. Between 30 and 45.

   C. Between 45 and 65.

   D. Over 65.

7. My weight is:

   A. Right where it should be for someone my age, gender, and height.

   B. I could stand to lose a few pounds.

   C. Mostly where it should be, when I don't eat during the day or when I use diet aids.

   D. Would be perfect if I were 6 inches taller.

8. I worry most about:

   A. Why worry?

   B. Just the glitches.

   C. Work, kids, retirement, my relationship, and money (or lack of).

   D. Everything.

Now add up your score. Give yourself 1 point for each A, 2 points for each B, 3 points for each C, and 4 points for each D. If you scored:

➤ Less than 10, your risk of heart problems is no higher than normal. You're feeding your heart well, keeping it in good shape through exercise, and heredity has been kind to you. Keep up the good work (and do an extra lap for us)!

➤ Between 11 and 15, you're taking unnecessary chances with your cardiac health. Take a look at the risk factors you can control, and make some heart-healthy changes in your life. Remember, improving your diet and increasing the amount of moderate exercise you get has the added benefit of weight control.

➤ Between 16 and 20, it's still not too late to change those risky behaviors. Consider swapping a few of those pizza nights for evenings playing basketball or dancing (aerobic, line, ballroom—whatever gets you moving). If you can't remember when you last had your blood cholesterol level and blood pressure checked, make an appointment to do so. Develop a heart-healthy diet and exercise plan with your doctor. If you smoke, stop.

➤ Higher than 20, yikes! You're living on the edge… and your sedentary ways are eroding it away. It's time for a heart-to-heart chat with your heart, which is probably sending signals you're ignoring (like getting winded when you bend down to tie your shoes…). You can still make a positive difference by changing your eating and exercise habits. Schedule an appointment with your doctor for a complete physical, then get started on your new heart-healthy life. It's worth the effort—you can do it, and you'll love the results!

What Every Woman Should Know

For all that women put up with for being women—like monthly mood swings and mid-life hot flashes—it seems only fair that we should get a break somewhere along the line. For a long time, we believed our break came with heart disease. Heart problems were men's problems, and our hormones sheltered us from them just as surely as they gave us the ability to bear children. Then along came the startling discovery that equality in other areas—job stress, smoking, poor dietary habits, and lifestyles made sedentary by machines—meant equality in the risk of heart disease, too. In 1990, equity passed a dubious milestone when 52 percent of deaths from heart disease occurred in women—the first time heart disease claimed more women than men. More than 10 million American women have some form of heart disease today—1 in 10 women between the ages of 45 and 64, and 1 in 4 over the age of 65. Women who have heart attacks are twice as likely to die as men who have heart attacks. Nearly 250,000 women will die from heart disease this year—far more than the number who will lose their lives to any kind of cancer.

Though heart disease has established itself as an equal-opportunity killer, it doesn't always look the same in women as in men. In men, the warning signs of a heart attack are classic and well-known: pressing or crushing chest pain; pain radiating to the arms, shoulders, and neck; sweating; nausea; and shortness of breath. While a woman having a heart attack may have these symptoms, she is just as likely to experience vague discomfort accompanied by a "feeling" that something is wrong. Listen to your body! If you experience two or more of the following symptoms, see your doctor immediately:

➤ Pain or heaviness in your chest that lasts more than a few minutes.

➤ "Indigestion" that doesn't go away with antacids.

➤ Unusual lightheadedness, dizziness, shortness of breath, or nausea.

➤ Tingling or pain in your arm, shoulder, or neck (especially on the left side of your body).

➤ A disconcerting sense that something is seriously wrong with the way your chest feels.

Don't think a heart attack can't happen to you because you're a woman—it can, and it does to half a million women each year. And don't be afraid to be specific, persistent, and frank with your doctor about your concerns if you think your doctor is brushing you off— ask for explanations when what you're hearing doesn't make sense. Not all doctors know that women's symptoms can be so different from men's or that heart disease is so prevalent in women today. Old habits die hard, even for doctors, and heart disease has been a man's problem for many years.

Just for YOU
When birth control pills first came out in the early 1970s, they contained relatively high doses of estrogen. This raised blood pressure and blood cholesterol levels in some women, which increased their risk of heart attack. Today's formulations have much lower estrogen doses and have very little effect on a woman's risk of heart attack.

Red Alert!
Women don't always experience "classic" symptoms when having a heart attack. If you are a woman age 40 or older, and you have two or more symptoms, especially during exercise, seek medical attention immediately.

Do Heart Problems Run in Your Family?

Genes give you more than blue eyes or long legs. Certain genes can predispose you to certain problems, such as diabetes and heart disease. Sometimes a child comes into this world with congenital heart problems, which are not necessarily genetic in nature but occur during development in the uterus. In genetic heart problems, which tend to manifest themselves in adulthood, there is often a strong family history. Certain proteins present in some people allow heart disease to develop earlier than is typical, often when no other risk factors are present.

This is not to say that just because Uncle Norbert had a heart attack when he was 42, you'll have early heart disease, too. Any number of other factors could have influenced Uncle Norbert's condition, including diet, a sedentary lifestyle, smoking, and borderline or undetected diabetes. These factors were everyday life for most Americans before we knew of their role in accelerating the course of heart disease, making it hard to know why Uncle Norbert had a heart attack as a young man. A genetics study would involve a detailed exploration of your family tree to determine whether patterns of heart disease exist. This is something you can do yourself as you gather health information about family members.

> **By Heart**
> *Congenital* heart problems are those present from birth. Most have nothing to do with genes but rather are malformations that occurred during development, and many are correctable through surgery. Heart problems are considered *genetic* when there is a strong family history. Genetic heart problems usually show up in adulthood.

Climbing Your Family Tree: Construct a Genogram

Does heart disease run in your family? Construct a quick genogram or family health tree to find out. Start by drawing a big tree on a piece of paper (be sure your paper's big enough to accommodate your extended family). Put your name on the trunk. Put the names of your brothers and sisters on the first branches coming off the trunk, then your mother's name and your father's name. Fill in the names of as many biological relatives as you know—grandparents, aunts, uncles, and cousins. If Aunt Sally went on medication for high blood pressure when she was 47 and Uncle Norbert died of a heart attack when he was 63, fill this in—add as much health information as you know about everyone, including dates and causes of death. Was Uncle Norbert overweight and a smoker? Did he have his first heart attack when he was 40? Remember to include this kind of related information as well. Update your genogram once a year or so, and take it with you to your doctor's appointment when you have a routine physical exam. The information can help your doctor determine whether you're at a higher risk for heart problems or other medical conditions.

> **Cardio Care**
> Confused about what family history matters? Follow the "speed limit" rule: Heart disease in men under 55 and women under 65 is what doctors consider a positive family history. Your grandfather's heart attack at age 82 not.

"It Doesn't Matter What I Do—I'm Doomed!"

Wrong! Even if every relative from the roots to the top branches of your family tree has had heart problems, you can still take action to minimize your chances of being next. Nature doesn't always win out over environment. The three most important things you can do are (come on, all together now):

➤ Eat right

➤ Exercise regularly

➤ Stop (or never start) smoking

If you maintain a healthy weight, your body is in good physical condition, and your blood cholesterol and blood pressure are normal, you can delay or even offset the potential risk factors you inherited. Remember, a risk factor is just a likelihood that a certain event will occur. You can't be certain when you step off a curb that a speeding car won't hit you. No matter what you do, you can't control that reckless driver. But you can reduce the likelihood that he or she will hit you. Stay in the crosswalk, cross with the light, and look in all directions before you leave the sidewalk. In the same way, you can reduce the risk factors that are within your control to lower your overall risk.

So all of you who have heart problems in your family tree, stand up. Put your right hand over your heart, and repeat after us: "I can do good things for my heart." Then read on, so you can learn more about what those good things are.

Just for YOU

African-Americans have a higher risk of hypertension and coronary heart disease than do individuals of other races/ethnicity. For example, African-American men are nearly four times more likely to die from high blood pressure than are white American men. African-American women between the ages of 35 and 74 are nearly 40 percent more likely to die from a heart attack than white American women in the same age range. Researchers don't fully understand why these differences exist; it seems to be a combination of genetic and lifestyle factors.

Take It to Heart

Are you an apple or a pear? Research shows that *where* you carry your body fat matters more than *how much* of it you're packing. People who carry their extra weight around their middles, the "apple" body shape, are more prone to heart disease than are people who bulk up through the hips, buttocks, and thighs—the "pear" body shape. Men are more likely to gain weight in an apple pattern, and women are more apt to take on the pear shape with weight gain.

You're Not Getting Any Younger

Sorry to remind you, but you're not getting any younger, which makes it all the more important that you listen to your heart. With aging come certain inevitable changes. Some are merely annoying (and funny when they happen to someone else)—body parts succumb to the influence of gravity, hair stops growing where you want it and sprouts where you don't, eyes refuse to focus on anything within arm's reach, "character" wrinkles propagate while you sleep. The process of aging starts with your first breath and doesn't end until your last. While you can't stop the process, you can take action to avoid aging before your time.

No one really knows why we age, though researchers know quite a bit about how. From about age 20 on, microscopic granular material begins to form in heart and nerve cells. The granules seem to be accumulations of molecular waste produced by your body's cells. Though a minor influence well past midlife, by age 80, the fat and connective tissue of this material can displace as much as 10 percent of the muscle fiber in the heart. The heart "flabs out" and becomes less efficient. Though your heart rate doesn't change much as you grow older (as long as you don't develop heart disease), the amount of blood the heart pumps with each beat lessens. Blood vessels thicken and become less elastic, too, which reduces their ability to flex and relax as your heart sends blood pulsing through them. The higher resistance sends signals to your heart to pump harder, gradually raising blood pressure. A normal blood pressure of 120/70 at age 25 can become 150/80 fifty years later.

The good news is that the effects of this and other aspects of aging are highly variable. A healthy body may function at age 80 like most bodies at age 40. As we learn more about the factors that shape how we age, we learn how to influence them. An American male born in 1900 had a life expectancy of just 48 years; one born in 1950 gained 18 years to age 66, and one born today can expect to live to age 73 (a woman, ages 51, 71 and 79, respectively). Researchers project that if we could eliminate heart disease, the number-one cause of death after age 65, life expectancy would increase by nearly 10 years for men and 12 years for women.

Teaching an Old Heart New Tricks

No matter how old your heart is, it will benefit from the heart-healthy changes you make in your life. Of course, it's not the same fresh, strong muscle it was when you were 20. After all, that fist-sized muscle in the center of your chest has worked hard since before your birth. The older your heart is, the more likely it has experienced some problems through the years.

But the heart has a remarkable capacity to compensate for enormous amounts of damage. Heart muscle tissue that dies during a heart attack or as the result of progressive heart disease is lost forever. Unlike liver tissue, the heart cannot regenerate itself. But other parts of the heart can take over for the damaged parts. Coronary arteries redirect themselves to diminish the blood supply to damaged parts of the heart and increase delivery to the sections that have picked up the load. Many people live reasonably normal lives after major heart attacks, in part because of medical treatments and technology and in part because they make changes in their diet and exercise habits. Attitude and state of mind are critical elements of the change process, too. You've got to "have heart" to make heart-healthy changes work.

The Least You Need to Know

➤ Risk factors for heart disease fall into two categories: risks you can eliminate through lifestyle changes and risks you're stuck with.

➤ Smoking is the most significant controllable risk factor for heart problems. Your body benefits within minutes when you stop smoking.

➤ Making lifestyle changes now to reduce your controllable risk factors lowers your risk of heart problems—no matter what your age or family history.

➤ Your risk of heart problems is higher if you are African-American, are over age 65, or have diabetes.

➤ Heart disease is now as common in women as it is in men. Both sexes need to think heart healthy.

➤ It's never too late to make heart-healthy lifestyle changes.

Part 2
How Do You Mend a "Broken" Heart?

"I feel as I always have, except for an occasional heart attack."

—Robert Benchley, as quoted by Groucho Marx

Now that you know how your heart works, you may wonder why it doesn't beat forever. The chapters in Part 2 take a look at what can go wrong with a heart, how your doctor determines what's happening with your heart, and what options modern medicine offers for fixing a "broken" heart.

Prevention remains the best cure. If your heart doesn't get sick, there's nothing to fix. When your heart needs help, technology makes possible procedures doctors dared not dream of 30 years ago. But keep your feet on terra firma. It's not the Star Trek generation yet. Recovery still requires active participation from you.

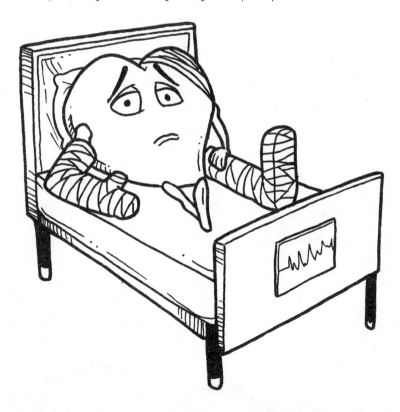

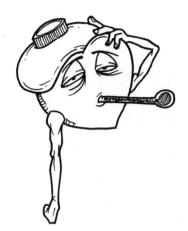

Chapter 5

Do You Feel Heart Sick?

In This Chapter

➤ Heart disease numbers and statistics

➤ Signs and symptoms of heart disease

➤ Communicating with your doctor

➤ Cardiopulmonary resuscitation (CPR)

Which do you fear more, cancer or heart disease? If you're like most Americans, you dread the "big C." Yet heart disease causes more deaths than cancer and the next six causes of death combined—nearly one of every two deaths in the United States today. More than one in five Americans (over 58 million) have some form of *cardiovascular disease* (CVD)—high blood pressure, coronary heart disease, stroke, or rheumatic heart disease. More than 2,600 of them die as a result each day—that's about one death every 33 seconds. The National Center for Health Statistics projects that eliminating heart disease would add ten years to life expectancy; eliminating all forms of cancer combined would add just three years.

So where's the good news in these bleak statistics? Sitting right in front of this book. You are the good news, because you have the ability to reduce your odds of being among them. Sure, your doctor and advances in medical technology could save your life if a cardiac crisis occurs. But you and you alone can make the lifestyle changes that can lower your risk of getting heart disease in the first place.

Take It to Heart

Not too fond of mornings? Your heart may share your aversion. Nearly half of all heart attacks occur between 6 a.m. and noon. Researchers aren't sure why this is, although they speculate that the mere process of waking up stresses the heart as it "gears up" to meet the needs of an active body.

How Are You Feeling Lately?

What's your body telling you these days? Does sprinting for the bus that's about to pull away leave you huffing and sweating? What does the body staring back at you from the mirror look like? Are you so exhausted at the end of the day that it takes all the energy you have left to collapse on the couch? Do these symptoms signal heart disease? Not always. Most people occasionally experience the feelings and discomforts typically associated with heart disease that are nothing more than the minor aches and pains that let us know we're alive. The good news is that simply adding some moderate exercise to your life can give you an energy and mood boost, as well as lower your blood pressure.

Red Alert!
Minutes matter during a heart attack. The risk of sudden cardiac death or ventricular fibrillation is greatest during the first five or six minutes. If your heart stops (which it doesn't always do during a heart attack), you have five minutes until brain death. If you think you're having a heart attack or you see someone who might be having a heart attack, don't wait. Summon help immediately!

Recognizing Signs and Symptoms

A heart attack happens in a finger-snap. One instant you're doing whatever you do in the course of your usual day, and the next you've got wires on your chest and needles in your arms. But should a heart attack come as a surprise? Not as often as it does. The events that set the stage for heart problems and a heart attack develop over years, even decades. Long before your heart breaks down, it sends you messages—some subtle, some pretty direct—to say, "Hey, wake up! I'm hurting in here!" Are you listening? You'd better be—your life depends on it!

Doctors consider certain warnings classic, though not conclusive, signs of heart trouble. **Though symptoms may differ among men and women, anyone can experience any symptom.** If you have any of these symptoms, have your doctor check them out.

Table 5.1 Possible Warning Signs of Heart Trouble

Symptom	For Men	For Women	Could Also Be
Pain	Sudden squeezing or pressure in chest; may radiate to shoulders and arms	Burning sensation in chest area; tingling in shoulders and arms	Ulcer, severe indigestion, gall-bladder problem, pulled or bruised chest wall muscle
Shortness of breath	Accompanying chest pain; with exercise or exertion	Feeling of breathlessness over several days or weeks, may wake up at night with sensation of being unable to breathe	Overexertion; lung problems; poor physical condition
Tiredness, lack of energy	All the time	All the time; sometimes overwhelming fatigue	Anemia, stress, various ailments
Swelling in hands and feet	Painless	Painless; may be more noticeable in the evening	Heat; in women, hormonal fluctuations; leg vein problem
Lightheadedness	May be accompanied by nausea, sweating	May be accompanied by nausea, fainting	

Notice that these symptoms can indicate problems other than heart disease; even chest pain can have any number of other causes. Only your doctor can help you sort out your symptoms and your risk factors. Many of us have a mental picture of the classic heart attack that happens when shoveling snow. But a heart attack is just as likely to happen while you're just reading the paper. Only half of all people experience a "precipitating" event such as exercise or stress.

The "Big One": Is It a Heart Attack?

Recognizing a heart attack, even when it's yours, can be difficult. Despite the common warning signs, no two heart attacks are the same. You might have excruciating chest pain… or none. You could feel like a giant hand has squeezed all the air out of your lungs… or like that pizza was just too spicy. The fact is, most people don't realize they're having a heart attack even while it's happening. And many who think they might be having a heart attack don't want to consider the possibility and insist that they're not.

So how do you know if this is The Big One? Quite simply, you don't. At the risk of boring you with repetition, we say again: *If you have any of the symptoms of heart attack, get thee to an emergency room. Now.* Not after you finish mowing the lawn, taking a shower, or cleaning the kitchen. (Yes, people having heart attacks really do these things before they

53

call for help.) While you're busy trying to tidy up, your life is slipping away. With each passing minute, more of your heart dies. Your odds of telling your grandchildren how you survived The Big One are immensely higher when you receive immediate treatment. More than 60 percent of those who die of a heart attack do so within the first hour, many before they get to the hospital. Who cares how your yard looks or that you left dirty dishes in the sink? Certainly not your family and friends who wish they were gathered around your hospital bed and not your casket! On the bright side, if you receive prompt care to minimize the damage to your heart, you could be back to your normal activities (even work) in three months.

It Can't Happen to Me!

Choose the reason you couldn't possibly have heart disease (go ahead, pick several if they apply):

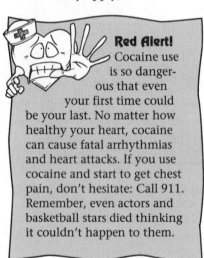

Red Alert! Cocaine use is so dangerous that even your first time could be your last. No matter how healthy your heart, cocaine can cause fatal arrhythmias and heart attacks. If you use cocaine and start to get chest pain, don't hesitate: Call 911. Remember, even actors and basketball stars died thinking it couldn't happen to them.

❑ I'm too young.

❑ My blood cholesterol level is good.

❑ I'm a woman.

❑ My blood pressure is normal.

❑ No one in my family has ever had heart disease.

❑ I'm in top physical condition.

❑ I haven't tasted French fries since I was 12.

❑ I'm too busy to have heart disease.

If you picked any of these, you couldn't be more wrong. Heart disease is an equal-opportunity killer. ANYONE can have heart disease, and ANYONE can die by ignoring its warning signs and symptoms.

The Troubled Heart

Like their risk factors, the various heart problems are often close cousins. *Angina pectoris* (heart-related chest pain) signals the presence of coronary artery disease, for example, and *myocardial infarction* (heart attack) represents an outcome. Congestive heart failure is the ultimate consequence of heart disease, usually an indication of long-term problems.

The damage heart disease causes is permanent. Once it happens, it doesn't go away, even if medication or surgery makes your symptoms disappear. The more damage your heart receives, the less able it is to sustain the lifestyle you want to live. This is why prevention is so critical—and the earlier you start, the better your chances of saving your heart. Symptoms are sometimes very subtle and easy to miss or ignore. By the time you discover you have heart disease, it could be too late. In as much as 30 percent of all heart disease, the first indication of a problem is sudden cardiac death—and half of those who die do so before they can get to a hospital.

Coronary Artery Disease: A Clog in the Plumbing

Two conditions contribute to *coronary artery disease* (CAD, also called *coronary heart disease*, or CHD): atherosclerosis and arteriosclerosis. When you enter this life, the inside walls of your arteries are smoother than the proverbial sitting end of your anatomy. Before long, the process of living leaves tiny deposits along those walls called *plaque*. These glue-like, microscopic collections of fatty substances and cellular debris cling to the smooth walls of your arteries. As the years go on, these deposits become large enough to restrict the flow of blood through your arteries (atherosclerosis).

At the same time, aging thickens and hardens the walls of your arteries, making them less flexible and increasing the effort your heart expends to move blood through them (arteriosclerosis). Eventually, it becomes difficult for blood to make it through the arteries at all; plaque may block an artery completely, or an artery may go into spasm. When this happens in the arteries that feed your heart, your heart doesn't get enough oxygen to fuel its needs. Doctors call this condition *myocardial ischemia*. And when your heart starves, it quits working.

Coronary artery disease often, though not always, warns you that it has a stranglehold on your heart. Shortness of breath with exercise or exertion, a dull pain in your chest or shoulders (angina), and lightheadedness are all warning signs. These signs may be vague, or you may have no inkling that you have CAD until it causes a heart attack. Treatment focuses on relieving the constrictions caused by atherosclerosis and may include balloon angioplasty or coronary bypass surgery, followed by a low-fat diet and increased exercise. Living a heart-healthy lifestyle before CAD starts is the best way to delay its effects until well into old age.

Cardio Care
An aspirin a day could keep a heart attack at bay. Aspirin has a mild blood-thinning effect that helps prevent clots from forming in your blood vessels. The American Heart Association recommends that if you've had a heart attack or you have heart disease, you take one baby aspirin (or one-half regular-strength adult aspirin) each day. Aspirin isn't for everyone, though. Talk with your doctor before using aspirin in this way.

Just for YOU
If you have diabetes, you face an increased risk for "silent" heart attack. While about 23 percent of heart attacks happen without pain in the general population, about 39 percent of heart attacks in people with diabetes send no warning. If you have diabetes, see your doctor regularly and pay attention to the "little" signs that could signal heart disease.

Angina Pectoris: Not Enough to Go Around

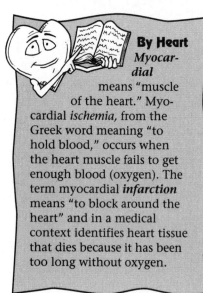

By Heart
Myocardial means "muscle of the heart." Myocardial *ischemia*, from the Greek word meaning "to hold blood," occurs when the heart muscle fails to get enough blood (oxygen). The term myocardial *infarction* means "to block around the heart" and in a medical context identifies heart tissue that dies because it has been too long without oxygen.

Angina is more of a symptom than a disease, an indication that you have CAD that shortchanges your heart's blood supply. Angina is the dull pain of your heart's complaint that it doesn't have enough oxygen. The most common form of angina occurs when you ask your heart to work harder, like during moderate to strenuous exercise or strong emotions. Running through the airport to catch your flight or down the street to catch your bus might trigger an angina attack, while walking at a regular pace wouldn't. Angina tells you that your heart is experiencing a temporary shortage of blood (oxygen) and usually goes away when your body returns to a state of rest. Doctors often treat angina with nitroglycerin or other medications to cause your arteries to expand, letting more blood through and relieving the pain. Angina is a sign that you are at increased risk for heart attack. Coronary artery spasms that temporarily reduce blood flow to the heart can cause a less common form of angina called *variant* or *Prinzmetal's angina*. Variant angina occurs without physical or emotional stress, often at night.

Myocardial Infarction: Heart Attack to You and Me

During a heart attack, a portion of your heart suddenly and permanently loses its blood supply, almost always as a result of CAD. The heart muscle in the affected area dies, and your heart can go into ventricular fibrillation (a rapid, useless fluttering), or sometimes your heart stops beating. If this happens, it causes cardiac arrest (sudden cardiac death). You also can experience a myocardial infarction and not know it if the affected area of your heart is small and your coronary arteries quickly compensate. The damage to your heart is permanent, however, and puts you at greater risk for other heart problems like arrhythmias, angina, and congestive heart failure. About two-thirds of those who have a heart attack survive, and many return to normal (and hopefully heart-healthier) lives.

Arrhythmias: Heart Out of Synch

Your heart's electrical system precisely synchronizes an amazing sequence of activity, day in and day out. Occasionally, problems interrupt your heart's synchronization and cause arrhythmias.

Arrhythmias can be primary electrical problems, arising from "shorts" in the sinoatrial node and other disruptions. Some people have accessory pathways, or "extra wiring," that lure electrical impulses off their regular routes. Coronary artery disease and damage from *myocardial infarctions* (MIs) can also cause arrhythmias. Remember, each fiber of your heart muscle conducts electrical impulses. When those fibers are damaged, as happens when CAD or an MI destroys sections of heart tissue, the disruption "breaks the circuit." Sometimes electrical impulses find their way around the disruption and continue the heart's beating without noticeable problems. More often, the impulses become confused when they encounter the disruption and either stop or disperse ineffectively through nearby tissues. Atrial fibrillation is a common arrhythmia. Without treatment, it increases your risk of stroke. Often, the only symptom of atrial fibrillation is an irregular pulse. If your pulse seems to beat irregularly, rather than steadily (especially if the rate is over 100), have your doctor check you out.

Take It to Heart

Many airlines that make long nonstop flights now carry defibrillators onboard and train flight attendants to use them to revive heart attack victims. Even in today's modern pressurized cabins, the atmosphere is like that in Denver, a mile above sea level. The thinner air has lower oxygen concentrations that can stress a weakened heart, especially one already feeling the strain of that mad dash to the gate to catch a flight about to leave without you.

Ventricular fibrillation is a particularly dangerous arrhythmia. This arrhythmia has no pattern whatsoever; your heart's ventricles beat wildly and rapidly without pumping any blood out. Your heart can only take this for a short time before it says "Enough!" and shuts down entirely. Ventricular fibrillation often accompanies a major myocardial infarction. Emergency personnel may use a defibrillator to deliver a brief shock to your heart. This momentarily stops all your heart's electrical impulses, which then resume in a regular rhythm. Other arrhythmias are less critical and disappear with medication.

Heart Murmurs: Valve Problems

A murmur sounds like such a gentle, soothing thing, doesn't it? In most situations, a mild heart murmur is nothing to worry about. Some murmurs are serious, sounding to your doctor more like the swan song of valve disease. Valves, you remember, are the gatekeepers of your heart's chambers. There are four (aortic, mitral, pulmonary, and tricuspid) that can malfunction, usually by failing to close properly. This

Just for YOU

Women are twice as likely as men to have mitral valve prolapse, or MVP. Your doctor may hear a heart click or murmur during a routine physical examination. In MVP, the mitral valve between the left atrium and the left ventricle fails to close properly. If you have MVP, you may get palpitations or funny chest pains (not serious). Most MVP is mild and requires no treatment, though may make you more susceptible to a heart valve infection. Your dentist may prescribe antibiotics before dental procedures as a preventive measure.

allows blood to "backwash" into the chamber that just pumped it out. Valves can also develop stenosis, which means the valve openings become narrow, preventing the chamber from pumping out its full volume of blood. Some valve problems are congenital (present from birth); reduced blood flow from CAD and damage from MIs can cause other valve problems. Surgery, including replacing the diseased valve with an artificial one, is often a successful treatment option.

Take It to Heart

Though Sir Alexander Fleming discovered the penicillin "magic bullet" in 1928, the antibiotic remained obscure until World War II brought a demand for its infection-fighting properties. Doctors soon realized that penicillin stopped other infections as well, including the dangerous childhood disease rheumatic fever, which causes serious damage to the heart valves. Today, rheumatic fever and its deadly consequences are rarely seen in developed countries.

Heart Failure: Supply-and-Demand Crisis

As this condition's name implies, the heart can no longer pump enough blood to meet the body's needs—demand exceeds supply. Sometimes called *congestive heart failure* (CHF), heart failure is a gradual and progressive disease that may take many years to reach the point of symptoms. Early symptoms are quite vague, ranging from mild swelling especially in the feet and ankles to breathlessness and fatigue. While these symptoms are classic, they are by no means unique to heart failure and may be misdiagnosed as other problems until their connection to the heart becomes obvious. The same risk factors that contribute to other forms of heart disease can lead to heart failure.

Just for YOU

Do you have diabetes? Your risk for heart failure is two to eight times that of someone who doesn't. The abnormal blood sugar levels common even in controlled diabetes weaken your heart muscle, making it vulnerable to heart failure. You can minimize your risk by keeping your diabetes and your other heart disease risk factors under strict control.

What to Do If You're Feeling Heartsick

What if you've reached this point in this book and you're saying to yourself, "Whoa, I think I have some of these symptoms!"? If you have significant risk factors, put down the book and pick up the phone. Schedule an immediate appointment with your doctor to evaluate your symptoms. If you know you have some risk factors but haven't had any symptoms that you know of, schedule an appointment for a routine physical exam, and plan to discuss your concerns with your doctor during your appointment.

Going to the Doctor

No matter how much you like your doctor, odds are that most times you leave the office after a visit with questions you forgot to ask. This time, sit down with a pen and a piece of paper before you go for your appointment (or now, while this is all fresh in your mind). Make a list of what concerns you. What questions do you have? Write down what you know about who had what and when they got it—your family's history with heart disease. Take your lists with you when you go for your appointment! (Your notes don't do you any good at home on the kitchen table.) Mark the most important two or three concerns with an asterisk (*); remember, your appointment will likely last 15 to 20 minutes. Ask questions about what's on your list and on your mind. When your doctor answers, take a few seconds to replay the response in your mind to be sure you understand it. If you don't, ask more questions.

Your doctor wants to discuss your concerns but unfortunately has only a limited time to spend with you. Being prepared helps you get the most from that time. Don't be afraid to be an educated health consumer. If you know that high blood pressure runs in your family, read up on it to gain a baseline understanding before you start asking your doctor questions. The more actively you participate in your health care, the more likely you are to follow your doctor's recommendations. After all, your health is your responsibility.

Cardio Care

Do you follow your doctor's advice? More than half of all people don't, either because they don't understand what they're supposed to do, or they don't understand why they're supposed to do it. When you go to the doctor, seek that understanding. Ask questions and seek participation in choosing treatment options. You'll feel better!

Is the Way You Live Helping or Hurting?

There's no doubt that advances in medical technology save hundreds of thousands of lives that otherwise would be lost to heart disease. It's easy and comforting to believe that your doctor and hospital can magically snatch you back from the hands of death when your heart reaches a state of crisis. We've come to expect immediate, positive results as we've become what sociologists call an *instant-gratification* society. Who wants to go home after a hectic day at work to face the day's most dreaded decision: what to have for dinner? We want what we want, now. Just stop at the drive-through and grab a burger and fries. And who has time to walk or bicycle to work, let alone jog or work out afterward?

What Else Could It Be?

Not all chest pains signal heart problems. In fact, a good many problems make themselves known through pain that seems to come from the chest—severe indigestion, ulcers and other stomach problems, muscle strains, lung problems, viruses, *pleurisy* (irritation of the tissue around the lungs), gallstones, and anxiety can make you think they're heart problems. Don't feel embarrassed if you go to your doctor, or even the hospital emergency room, with "chest" pain only to find out that its source is something else. In all likelihood, that something else is a problem that needs medical attention, too. The adage "better safe than sorry" couldn't be more true. Consider the experience a reminder of how important your heart health is.

In an Emergency: Jump-Start a Heart

When your heart stops, it doesn't take long for the rest of you to follow. Without the blood your heart pumps, your body can't function. Here's a timeline for what happens when you have a heart attack:

> First 5 minutes: Highest likelihood of sudden death
>
> First 15 minutes: Best time to call 911 and save your life
>
> First 24 hours: Best chance for blood-thinning medications (thrombolytics) to save your heart muscle
>
> First 2 days: Most important to be in the hospital because of the high risk of arrhythmia
>
> First 6 months: Best time to recover to your post–heart attack health

Do yourself a favor and enroll your family in *cardiopulmonary resuscitation* (CPR) classes (especially if anyone in your family has heart disease). Most communities offer CPR classes free or at minimal cost through agencies like local health departments, fire or public safety departments, hospitals and medical centers, and chapters of organizations like the American Red Cross and the American Heart Association. It takes just a few hours of training to learn how to revive someone who has suffered cardiac arrest (cessation of heartbeat and breathing).

You can't learn CPR by just reading about it! Though we'll briefly discuss the procedures for this emergency life-saving technique, you must take classes to learn how to do chest compressions. If other people are around, shout out "Heart attack!" and ask for someone to call for emergency aid (911 in most communities in the United States). If you haven't taken a CPR class, make it a priority to sign up for one.

CPR for Adults

First, call or send someone for help. Then make sure the person is in cardiac arrest. Check for signs of breathing and a pulse.

To begin CPR, follow these steps:

➤ Place the person on his or her back on a hard, flat surface (the floor is ideal).

➤ Tip the head back so the chin juts up (the mouth should fall open).

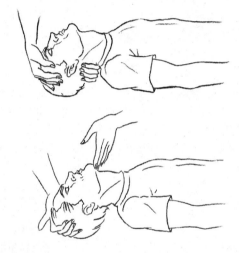

➤ Pinch the nose shut, take a deep breath, place your mouth over the victim's mouth, and blow.

➤ Wait 10 seconds to see if the person begins breathing. If not, give another breath and then begin cardiac compressions.

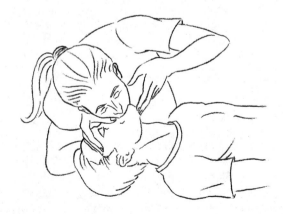

61

➤ Place the heel of your hand in the middle of the breastbone, then place the heel of your other hand over the back of your hand.

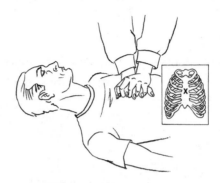

➤ Lock your elbows to keep your arms straight. Press down quickly and forcefully so the breastbone depresses 1¹/₂ to 2 inches, then release.

➤ Do this at a rate of 80 compressions per minute if you are alone, giving two breaths after every 15 compressions. If there are two of you, one should do the breathing and the other the compressions at a rate of one breath every five compressions.

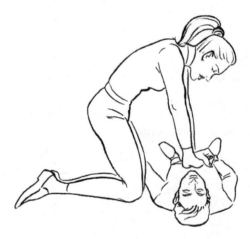

CPR for Children

Most kids stop breathing from choking, asthma, or infections, which in turn causes the heart to stop. It's very rare for a child to have a heart problem that would cause cardiac arrest unless it's congenital. Be especially alert to the possibility that the child is choking. Turn the child on its side and clap sharply on the back to dislodge any material. Do NOT put your finger in the mouth, since this might push a foreign object farther down the child's throat.

CPR for a child requires far less pressure during chest compressions and a more rapid rate. First call or send someone for help. Listen and watch for breathing, and feel for a pulse.

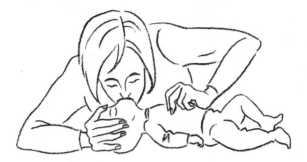

To administer CPR to a child, follow these steps:

➤ Place the child on his or her back on a hard, flat surface (like a table or the floor).

➤ Tip the head back so the chin juts up.

➤ Take a deep breath. For an infant, cover the mouth and nose with your mouth and blow. For an older child, pinch the nostrils and blow into the mouth. Do this twice.

➤ Wait 10 seconds to see if the child begins breathing. If not, start cardiac compressions.

➤ For an infant or small child, place two fingertips in the center of the breastbone. Press quickly, with enough force to depress the breastbone 1 to 1½ inches, and release.

➤ Do compressions at a rate 80 to 100 per minute. Breathe every third compression.

Remember: CPR is an emergency life-saving technique only! It's critical to get professional medical attention as quickly as possible.

The Least You Need to Know

➤ Treatment has come a long way in recent years, but preventing heart problems is still a better route to a long and productive life than fixing them.

➤ Heart problems often compound each other, just as risk factors do.

➤ Write down your concerns and questions before you go to the doctor so that you won't forget them.

➤ CPR saves lives. If you don't already know CPR, enroll in a class to learn it.

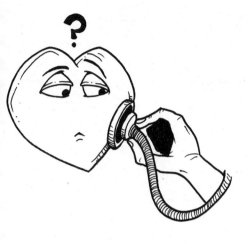

Straight to the Heart

So your genogram (family history) turned up a trend of heart disease on your mother's side of the family? Pizza, cheeseburgers, omelets, and milkshakes form your basic food groups? Grocery shopping on Saturday morning is your idea of a marathon? Schedule that physical exam! (If you have more urgent symptoms, like chest pain or difficulty breathing, see your doctor right away.) It's time to find out what's going on with your heart.

While your concerns are fresh in your mind, take a few minutes to jot them down. This outline can help you organize your thoughts.

These relatives had heart problems before age 55 (men) or age 65 (women):

Name/Relationship	Heart Problem	Age at Diagnosis	Result
_____	_____	_____	_____
_____	_____	_____	_____
_____	_____	_____	_____

I am concerned about my risk for heart disease because: _____

_____

I already have these health conditions:

Health Condition	When Diagnosed	Treatment/Medication
_____	_____	_____
_____	_____	_____
_____	_____	_____

My last blood cholesterol level was _____, taken in _____.

Other questions I have for my doctor: _____

_____

Your list might look something like this:

These relatives had heart problems before age 55 (men) or age 65 (women):

Name/Relationship	Heart Problem	Age at Diagnosis	Result
Norbert; dad's brother	Heart attacks	52	Died of heart attack at 63
Sally; mom's sister	High blood pressure	47	Takes medication

I am concerned about my risk for heart disease because: <u>I get winded when I have to walk up more than one flight of stairs, and I know I don't eat right. Sometimes I feel my heart flutter.</u>

I already have these health conditions:

Health Condition	When Diagnosed	Treatment/Medication
Underactive thyroid	3 years ago	Take levothyroxine 0.25mg every morning

My last blood cholesterol level was <u>I don't know</u>, taken in <u>I've never had one done.</u>

Other questions I have for my doctor: <u>Should I be drinking a glass of wine a day to prevent heart disease?</u>

Remember to take your notes with you for your appointment and a pen or pencil so you can write down what your doctor tells you.

Take It to Heart

For centuries, doctors seldom touched their patients. Doctors relied on what they could see and what their patients said. Austrian physician Leopold Auenbrugger (1722–1809) broke with tradition when he developed a procedure he called "chest percussion" to reveal medical conditions within the chest. He tapped various locations on the chest with his finger, then listened to the sounds. Areas containing fluid had different sounds than those containing air. The method failed to catch on, since most doctors lacked the keen ear Dr. Auenbrugger possessed—he happened to be a musician as well. Doctors today sometimes use percussion to aid in diagnosing certain conditions that produce unique sounds, often using a stethoscope to help them hear.

Tests, Tests, and More Tests...

Depending on your age, apparent physical condition, family history, symptoms, and your doctor's instincts, you can expect some basic tests:

➤ Blood pressure

➤ Pulse and respiration (breathing) rate

➤ Auscultation (doctor listens to your heart and lungs using a stethoscope)

➤ Blood cholesterol level (and possibly blood triglyceride level); usually every five years after age 35 and more frequently if your results are abnormal

➤ Medical history

Nearly all visits to the doctor start with a blood pressure check. This simple test is quick, easy, and often identifies high blood pressure before it becomes a problem. Since high blood pressure seldom shows any sign of its presence until it causes a catastrophe like a stroke or heart attack, routine blood pressure screening is essential and effective.

Typically, a nurse or medical technician takes your blood pressure and counts your pulse and respirations (breathing rate) at the beginning of your visit. Your doctor will usually begin by talking with you about the reason for your visit and any health problems you've had in the past (doctors call this "taking a history"). Next you'll meet the cold end of a stethoscope, which

Cardio Care

Your blood pressure reading is most accurate when you are calm and relaxed, which isn't usually how you're feeling when you're in the doctor's office. If your reading is high or significantly different from earlier readings, ask your doctor to take your blood pressure again at the end of your visit.

your doctor places in various locations on your chest and back, listening to your heart and lungs. Finally, your doctor may order a blood cholesterol level.

Sometimes your doctor will order additional tests, particularly if your symptoms or family history hint at possible heart problems or you already have a diagnosis of heart disease. Some tests, like chest x-rays, are familiar and quick. Others use the latest technology to look inside your body without actually entering it. Often, you'll schedule these tests for another visit and possibly at another location like a local hospital. Some tests require special equipment, procedures, and a specially trained staff, so your doctor will ask you to schedule those separately from your visit.

Take It to Heart

A Dutch physiologist, Willem Einthoven (1860–1927), developed the first reliable electrocardiograph in 1903. Though electricity was still a novelty that had not yet invaded everyday life, the tiny volts that charged through the human heart intrigued Einthoven. His continued research to identify and chart the regular patterns of the heart's electrical activity earned him the 1924 Nobel Prize in physiology.

By Heart

Which is it, ECG or EKG? Either, though ECG is becoming the standard. The letters are an abbreviation for *ElectroCardioGram,* the name of the test that produces tracings of your heart's electrical activity. The process of performing an ECG is called *electrocardiography,* which means "electric heart writing." The abbreviation EKG comes from the German spelling that Einthoven and others used.

ECG: Take Me to Your Leader

Did you know your heart's an artist? Using the electrical impulses that regulate your heart's function (and with a little help from technology), it can "draw" a picture of its well-being. During a procedure called an *electrocardiography* (an ECG or EKG), electrodes that are attached to your chest, wrists, and ankles "pick up" the impulses and transmit them via wires called *leads* to a machine that records on paper the patterns of the impulses. The jagged peaks and valleys might look more like a bad week in the stock market to you, but to your doctor, the squiggles present an amazing image of your heart at work. Your doctor may order an ECG as a baseline (to establish a view of your healthy heart) or as a diagnostic aid to confirm or rule out suspicions of heart disease.

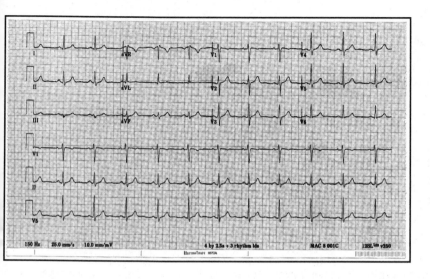

A normal ECG reading for a fifty-four-year-old Caucasian male.

Vent Rate: 68 bpm
PR interval: 150ms
QRS duration: 98ms
QT/QTc: 378/402ms
P-R-T axes: 58 16 50

Normal sinus rythm
Normal ECG

Courtesy University of Washington Medical Center

Exercise Tolerance ECG: Take a Walk on the Treadmill

A regular, or resting, ECG only shows what your heart's up to when it's not working very hard. Many symptoms of heart problems, like angina, only show up under stress. An exercise tolerance ECG records your heart's activity while you walk on a treadmill. You'll start out slow and level, like a stroll around the block. Since the purpose is to put some stress on your heart by making it work harder, the technician will gradually increase the treadmill's speed and angle. All the while, the technician keeps a close eye on what your heart's doing by watching the ECG as it records your heart's electrical impulses. You can stop the test any time if you experience chest pain, difficulty breathing, or feel too tired to continue. It's important to really push yourself, though, so the test gives an accurate picture of your heart when it works hard. Wear loose-fitting clothing and comfortable shoes that you can jog or run in when you go for your exercise tolerance ECG.

Abnormal results often indicate coronary artery disease. Under stress, your heart's arteries can't supply your heart with enough oxygen-carrying blood—a situation your heart complains about by sending odd electrical messages. You might feel a bit tired after an exercise tolerance ECG, especially if you don't get much exercise in your everyday life. Otherwise, the test causes no

Cardio Care
Have you had a heart attack or told that you have a heart rhythm problem? Ask your doctor for a representative ECG "strip" that you can carry with you when you travel. Then if you have any problems while you're away from home and your regular doctor, you can show the strip to the doctor who treats you. This can help doctors determine whether there is new damage to your heart.

Just for YOU
Women are more likely to have false positive results with exercise tolerance ECG testing. This indicates coronary artery disease when there is none. Researchers don't fully understand why this is. Your doctor may do additional tests if your results are positive just to be sure.

discomfort. It generally takes about half an hour (about 10 minutes actually on the treadmill) to complete. Your doctor may order an exercise tolerance ECG to evaluate chest pain, particularly "funny" chest pain that doesn't really fit a classic coronary artery disease pattern.

Holter Monitor: The Beat Goes On

Sometimes it's necessary to monitor your heart over a longer period of time. The Holter monitor, or ambulatory ECG, allows your doctor to record your heart's activity for 24 hours at a time. Wires connect five electrodes on your chest to a portable device similar to a cassette tape recorder in both size and function. The wires feed your heart's electrical impulses into the device, which records them on a slow-moving cassette tape. When you return after 24 hours, your doctor removes the electrodes and sends the tape to the ECG lab, where a technician transfers the information it contains to a paper printout. A Holter monitor is especially helpful for diagnosing transient symptoms (those that come and go without any predictability) like rhythm problems, atrial fibrillation, and angina.

When wearing a Holter monitor, you'll need to write down your daily activities on a log sheet. Your physician will match your activities with the 24-hour ECG printout to see what your heart's been doing all day.

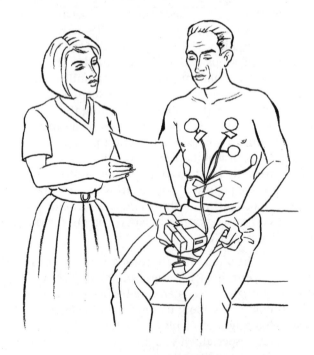

Echocardiography: Your Heart on Video

When most people think *ultrasound*, they think baby. Sound waves bounced through the lower abdomen produce pictures of the unborn baby, giving expectant parents (and doctors) their first glimpse of the newest family member. The same technology also gives doctors a way to see the heart in action without entering the chest. Sound waves bounce from different densities of tissue to produce images, or echoes, that show doctors each part of the heart—chambers, valves, and major vessels.

After applying a thin layer of a lubricating gel to your skin, a technician moves a *transducer* across your chest and left side. Remember those flip books with a slightly different picture on each page? One at a time, the images made little sense. But when you flipped the pages really fast, you got the whole picture, animated for your viewing pleasure. A computer compiles the ultrasound's images on videotape, producing a high-tech "flip book" featuring a complete two-dimensional moving picture.

Your doctor may order an echocardiogram to evaluate physical or structural abnormalities of your heart, like congenital heart disease, valve problems, major vessel abnormalities (particularly an aneurysm, a bulge resulting from vessel wall thinning), and heart muscle damage from myocardial infarction (heart attack).

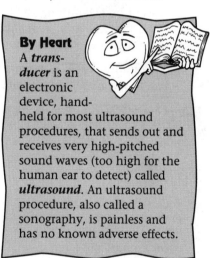

By Heart
A *transducer* is an electronic device, handheld for most ultrasound procedures, that sends out and receives very high-pitched sound waves (too high for the human ear to detect) called *ultrasound*. An ultrasound procedure, also called a sonography, is painless and has no known adverse effects.

If you fly a lot, you may know about Doppler radar for detecting dangerous wind-shear conditions at airports—those sudden, powerful down drafts that can slam a jet trying to land or take off into the ground like a child throwing a toy. That same technology, called the Doppler effect, can also measure how fast your blood shoots through the valves in your heart. Doppler echocardiography helps doctors assess how fast blood flows through abnormal heart valves and how turbulent that flow is. While regular echocardiography gives a good picture of your heart's structural integrity, adding Doppler gives the procedure another dimension. Your doctor may order a Doppler echocardiogram to evaluate valve disease and certain congenital heart disorders.

EBCT: "Ultrafast" CT Scanning for Early Disease Detection

Computerized tomography (CT) scans have come a long way since this high-tech combination of x-rays and computers made its debut in 1972. The most recent incarnation of this ubiquitous technology is the "ultrafast" CT scan, or *electron beam computed tomography* (EBCT). EBCT, like blood cholesterol level, is primarily valuable for its ability to predict your risk for developing coronary artery disease. EBCT measures the calcium level in the plaque that builds up in your coronary arteries. The higher the calcium level, the thicker the layer of plaque.

Your doctor may order an EBCT if you have a number of risk factors that place you at increased risk for coronary artery disease, such as a positive family history in combination with high blood cholesterol or blood pressure and angina, for example. Your doctor may also order an EBCT if you've had coronary bypass surgery or to evaluate how effectively your heart's chambers work.

Some researchers believe EBCT offers such promise for detecting coronary artery disease before it causes symptoms that they advocate its use as a screening tool. Others, including the American Heart Association, believe more studies are necessary to determine what difference this relatively expensive new technology can make in deciding treatment recommendations.

Nuclear Imaging: Radionuclides for Health

Your body continuously metabolizes various elements, such as oxygen, nitrogen, and carbon. Attaching *radionuclides* to these elements allows doctors to watch how quickly body tissues consume them. This shows whether the tissue is healthy or diseased.

Common nuclear imaging tests for the heart include *positron emission tomography* (PET) and *single photon emission computerized tomography* (SPECT). These tests involve injecting a tiny amount of *radionuclides*, like thallium-201 or Tc-99m sestamibi, into your vein. Don't worry, you won't glow in the dark—or even feel anything except the slight prick of the injection. After the radionuclides have been in your system long enough to reach your heart (usually within a few minutes), you lay on a table that enters a scanner. Shaped like a large donut, the scanner bounces energy impulses at your body. The impulses react with the energy the isotopes release; a computer collects these impulses and translates them into visual images.

By Heart
Radionuclides are radioactive substances that enter your body through injection or swallowing. Their radioactivity causes them to release particles of energy. Sophisticated scanning technologies track these particles as they enter various body tissues. Radionuclides leave your body in a few days and have no known side effects.

Your doctor may order cardiac nuclear imaging to detect suspected heart disease before it damages your heart or to confirm a need for coronary bypass surgery. Nuclear imaging procedures require expensive, sophisticated equipment and highly trained nuclear radiologists and often are available only in larger cities.

MRI: Magnet Power

Magnetic resonance imaging (MRI) uses bursts of magnetic energy to create high-contrast pictures of your heart, its blood vessels, and your blood as it flows through. There are no x-rays or radioactive materials. The powerful magnetic field the scan generates can affect pacemakers, hearing aids, and other objects (take off your watch, and leave your credit cards at home!). As a new and highly sophisticated technology, MRI remains quite expensive and continues to evolve as researchers refine its uses. Your doctor may order an MRI scan if you have a rare heart condition or if other procedures fail to provide clear information about a suspected problem with your heart.

Cardiac Catheterization: Are You Blocked?

During cardiac catheterization, doctors use the natural highway of your veins to thread a small tube, or catheter, into the arteries around your heart. After giving you medication to sedate you and injecting the skin surface with a local anesthetic, your doctor makes a tiny incision over a large vein like the femoral vein in your groin and slowly advances the catheter up to your heart. Through the catheter, your doctor can measure blood flow and oxygen levels, and also inject a liquid dye to make your coronary arteries visible using fluoroscopy (high speed x-ray movies). This shows where and to what extent plaque blocks your coronary arteries.

Your doctor may order cardiac catheterization after other tests (such as exercise tolerance ECG and echocardiogram) show that you have coronary artery disease. Cardiac catheterization results help your doctor decide which course of treatment is most appropriate for you. You may spend the night in the hospital following your catheterization just to make sure you don't experience any complications.

Why Doesn't My Doctor Order All the Latest Wonder-Tests?

If it's new, is it better? In some circumstances, certainly, but not always. Doctors consider several factors when deciding which tests to order. First and foremost, doctors want tests that will show them the information they're looking for—what's going on with your heart. The latest isn't always the greatest; some high-tech, high-cost procedures don't reveal any more information than the standard procedures doctors have used for years.

Second, your doctor wants information at minimal risk to you. Many diagnostic procedures come with a risk, very slight for most people, that they will cause the very problem they seek to diagnose. An exercise tolerance ECG can create ideal conditions for a heart attack, for example (though the risk of something this serious happening is extremely small—about 1 in 20,000). For most people, the benefit of knowing what's going on beneath those protective ribs is worth the slight risk of finding out more than you wanted to know. Other procedures have greater risks that your doctor must balance with the potential benefits. One risk of cardiac catheterization is heart attack or stroke from arterial plaque that the catheter dislodges as it enters your arteries. Of course, highly trained staff and special equipment are always at the ready to treat any problems that arise.

We talk about potential risks not to alarm you but to remind you that you are ultimately responsible for decisions involving your healthcare. It's very easy just to do what the doctor suggests; after all, you go to the doctor because he or she knows more than you do. A good reality check is the "Gee whiz" test. If your doctor says, "Gee whiz, it'd sure be nice to see this from another angle," ask what additional information this other angle will provide. The answer should offer a clear benefit. The "Gee whiz" test works from the other side, too. Today's media reports every scientific study and new technology. To fit into the sound-bite nature of news broadcasts and even newspaper articles, these reports often present highlights that will draw a listener's or reader's attention. The rest of the story is usually far less sensational. Yes, new technologies save lives. So do "old" ones.

The third factor doctors consider is cost-effectiveness—which tests give the most effective and efficient results? Technology gives us extraordinary opportunities to look inside the heart that otherwise would be impossible without surgery (or, not so long ago, not until an autopsy). These opportunities often come with extraordinary price tags, too. While you may think this doesn't matter to you because your insurance picks up the tab, the costs of healthcare affect us all. More and more health plans require you to pay a portion of your healthcare expenses. If you're retired or not working, you may not have private insurance. What do you think these common diagnostic procedures cost? The answers may surprise you.

Table 6.1 Typical Costs for Diagnostic Procedures

Fasting lipid panel (cholesterol and triglycerides)	$45
Standard ECG	$45
Exercise tolerance ECG	$310
24-hour Holter monitor	$250–300
Echocardiogram	$500–1,000
Nuclear imaging	$1,500
Cardiac catheterization	$4,300

Source: University of Washington

What Women Need to Know

A woman's body differs from a man's body, in obvious as well as subtle ways. These differences can matter when it comes to testing for heart problems. Certain anatomical attributes become liabilities when it comes to accurate test results. Large breasts and breast implants can reduce the diagnostic accuracy of echocardiography and nuclear imaging tests, as can obesity (in men as well as women). Women have a greater tendency to have false positive results with exercise tolerance ECG testing, as we mentioned earlier. Is driving a car with a clutch your daily exercise? If your lifestyle is sedentary, you're more likely to end an exercise tolerance ECG before it provides diagnostic results. This may make other, often invasive, testing necessary.

The bottom line for women: Talk with your doctor very specifically about gender differences in any tests he or she is considering, and ask for a full explanation of test results.

The Least You Need to Know

➤ An old-fashioned diagnostic tool—listening to your health history—leads doctors to many diagnostic determinations.

➤ The "latest and greatest" technology isn't necessarily appropriate for your symptoms and condition. Sometimes simple is better (and safer).

➤ Learn as much as you can about the tests your doctor orders and what the results mean.

➤ Test results differ between men and women, with women more likely to have false positives that require further investigation.

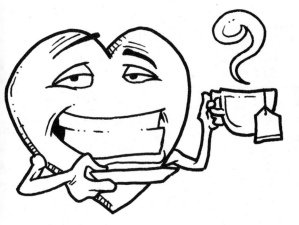

Rx: Heart Health

There are three general approaches to treatment for heart problems:

➤ Lifestyle changes

➤ Medications

➤ Interventional procedures

For most people, a total treatment plan combines at least two and sometimes all three of these approaches.

Drugs That Help Your Heart

For many heart problems, treatment is just a swallow away. Medications can lower blood pressure, strengthen the contracting power of your heart, control arrhythmias, and reduce blood cholesterol levels. When combined with lifestyle changes like increased physical activity and improved diet, medications can keep heart disease at bay for years. Medications that help your heart can be preventive, therapeutic (treatment), or a little of

Cardio Care
Make a list of the medications you take, the dosages or amount, and the time you usually take them. Carry the list with you, so if you need medical care, you or someone else can let the treating doctor know what you're taking.

both. Cholesterol-lowering medications are preventive, prescribed to reduce the likelihood that high blood cholesterol levels will cause a heart attack. (We discuss these medications in Chapter 14, "How Does Cholesterol Count?") Blood pressure medications are both preventive and therapeutic—they lower blood pressure, reducing the risk of stroke and heart attack. Some people with high blood pressure or heart failure also take drugs called *diuretics*, which lower blood pressure by removing extra fluid from your body to prevent further problems. Other drugs help restore heart functions to as normal as possible in the presence of heart disease.

Many heart medications are quite expensive, particularly the newer ones. Ask your doctor to explain medication choices. Your doctor will usually prescribe generic drugs (the same active ingredients without the costly name brand), which are less expensive. Some medications, particularly new ones, are not available in a generic form. Do you take medication for heart problems, high cholesterol, or high blood pressure? *How* do you take it? Be honest, now!

A. With rare exceptions, I take my pills according to the label directions.

B. I'm pretty good about taking my pills like I'm supposed to, though sometimes I forget a dose.

C. I take my pills like I'm supposed to when I can afford to buy them.

D. I don't like the side effects, so I don't take my pills very regularly.

E. I don't know why I have to take these blasted pills. What my doctor tells me doesn't make any sense, but if I ask questions, my doctor will think I'm stupid.

Red Alert!
Never stop taking medication for high blood pressure without first consulting your doctor! Suddenly stopping your medication can cause your blood pressure to shoot up, putting you at risk for stroke, heart failure, and heart attack. Once you start taking medication for your blood pressure, you'll probably take it for the rest of your life.

In reality, more than half of people don't take medications like they're supposed to. If you answered A or B, you're doing well and probably getting the full benefit of your medications. If you answered C, D, or E, it's time to talk with your doctor. Don't worry, your doctor won't think you're whining or stupid! Sometimes adjusting your dose, the time of day you take your medication, or even changing the medication can reduce or end side effects that bother you (though often side effects go away in a few weeks after your body has a chance to adjust to the medication). If you can't afford your medications, your doctor can help you find a solution—sometimes a less expensive medication will work, or there might be programs in your community that can help you out.

It's very important for you to take medications for your heart or blood pressure as your doctor instructs, at generally the same time each day, to maintain a constant level of the medication in your system. Ask your doctor or pharmacist what to do if you miss a dose. When C, D, or E describes how you take your medications, you're not getting the full benefits of them. Your doctor might unnecessarily increase your dose or add other medications because he or she is not seeing the results expected.

Table 7.1 Common Cardiac Drugs

Drug	Action	Prescribed to Treat
ACE inhibitors (angiotensin-converting enzyme)	Make the heart's work easier by blocking chemicals that constrict capillaries	High blood pressure, heart failure, after a heart attack
Anticoagulants (coumarin, aspirin)	Prevent clots from forming	After a heart attack or stroke
Beta blockers	Reduce the rate and force of heart's pumping action to reduce its oxygen needs	Angina, arrhythmias, high blood pressure (also migraines and glaucoma)
Calcium channel blockers	Slow movement of calcium across membranes of heart muscle cells to slow their contraction	Angina, arrhythmias, high blood pressure
Digitalis compounds (digoxin, digitoxin)	Regulate heart rate and strength of beat	Heart failure, arrhythmias
Diuretics ("water pills")	Reduce blood volume	High blood pressure, heart failure
Vasodilators (nitroglycerin)	Relax arteries	Angina, high blood pressure

There are dozens of different medications available to treat various kinds of heart disease, with new ones being discovered all the time. We've included brief descriptions of the ones doctors use most often. Doctors may prescribe these medications in combination with other drugs to treat multiple symptoms. Sometimes your body becomes resistant to a particular drug's effects, so your doctor will try something different. In general, it's best to stay with what works for as long as it works well for you rather than jumping to every new (and expensive) drug that comes out. Many newer medications don't achieve results different from current drugs; they just get the results in different ways.

ACE Inhibitors: Reducing Resistance

ACE inhibitors work to relax your blood vessels and reduce your heart's workload. ACE stands for *angiotensin-converting enzyme*, which causes your capillaries to constrict. "Inhibitor" means these drugs prevent this enzyme, which your kidneys produce, from working. ACE inhibitors work especially well for those who have high blood pressure in combination with diabetes or heart failure.

Your doctor may prescribe an ACE inhibitor along with a diuretic. Side effects can include dizziness, loss of appetite, rash, itching, and a slight dry cough. Newer drugs with similar actions, called angiotensin II receptor blockers, which seem to have fewer side effects, are also available. Common ACE inhibitors are captopril, enalapril, and lisinopril, under various brand names. Because these drugs are very expensive, your doctor may try other medications first.

Red Alert!
Do you take products containing acetaminophen (Tylenol is a common and familiar brand)? Many cold remedies include this drug in their ingredients to relieve fever and aches. Some studies show that acetominophen can interfere with anticoagulants, such as warfarin, by enhancing their effect. If you're taking anticoagulants (blood thinners), talk with your doctor or pharmacist before taking any medications that have acetaminophen in them.

Anticoagulants: Stopping Clots

Also called *blood thinners*, anticoagulant medications help keep your blood from forming clots. They don't actually cause your blood to become "thinner." This nickname refers to the thickened appearance of blood that is just beginning to clot, an action anticoagulants prevent.

Your doctor may prescribe an anticoagulant if you've just had a surgical procedure like coronary bypass or valve replacement. Heparin is a common anticoagulant you might receive by injection through an IV or subcutaneously (into the fatty tissue just under your skin). Anticoagulants you might take by mouth include dicoumarol and warfarin, under various brand names.

Aspirin also has a mild anticoagulating effect. The American Heart Association recommends a half aspirin a day (or a whole baby aspirin) *if you're not taking any other anticoagulants*. Always ask your doctor before taking aspirin in this way, and avoid aspirin-containing products if you're taking a prescription anticoagulant.

Beta Blockers: Easing Your Heart's Workload

Beta blockers act on your body's *neurotransmitters* (chemicals your nerve endings release). Beta blockers slow your heart rate and make your heart's contractions less forceful, reducing your heart's workload. Your doctor may prescribe a beta blocker if you have angina, arrhythmias, high blood pressure, heart failure, or have had a heart attack. Doctors also use beta blockers to treat migraine headaches and glaucoma.

Beta blockers can cause impotence in some men; if you experience this side effect, let your doctor know. There are likely other drugs your doctor can try to achieve the desired results. Common beta blockers include nadolol, propranolol, acebutolol, metoprolol, and carvedilol.

Calcium Channel Blockers: Slowing Heart Muscle Cells

Calcium channel is the medical term for the way the muscle cells in your heart and your arteries use calcium to move the electrical impulses that cause those cells to contract. When you take a drug that blocks some of this action, those cells don't contract quite so force-fully. This causes your arteries and heart to relax a bit, which lowers your blood pressure and improves blood flow.

Your doctor may prescribe a calcium channel blocker if you have high blood pressure, angina, or arrhythmias—often in combination with a diuretic or another medications. Common calcium channel blockers include diltiazem, nicardipine, nimodipine, and verapamil. Because these drugs are relatively new, most are available only as brand names and are expensive. If a less expensive medication has the same likelihood of bringing your symptoms under control, your doctor will probably try it first.

Red Alert!
Hold the grapefruit juice if you take calcium channel blockers! This otherwise healthful citrus drink appears to interfere with your liver's ability to metabolize these medications, which can lead to toxic blood levels. Ask your doctor or pharmacist if your medication is a calcium channel blocker and what other interactions present possible risks.

Digitalis Compounds: Keeping the Pace

Ancient doctors sometimes had their patients drink a tea made from the purple leaves of the foxglove plant to treat heart problems. The plant's digitalis compounds (digitoxin and digoxin), which today come from a laboratory rather than nature, strengthen and regulate your heartbeat. Your doctor may prescribe one of these drugs if you have arrhythmias or heart failure.

When you first start taking digoxin or digitoxin, your doctor will order regular blood tests to check the level of drug in your system. There's a fine line between therapeutic and toxic levels with digitalis compounds, and your doctor wants to be sure you stay on the right side of it. These drugs also interact with numerous other medications, so talk with your doctor or pharmacist before taking anything not prescribed for you, including over-the-counter medications.

Diuretics: Water Control

Diuretics tell your kidneys to pull more fluid from your blood and get rid of it. This reduces both blood pressure and *edema* (swelling in places like your ankles and feet). There are three kinds of diuretics, classified according to how they affect your kidneys: thiazide, loop, and potassium-sparing. Often, potassium, a vital electrolyte that plays a role in the electrical impulses that regulate your heartbeat, leaves with the fluid.

Your doctor may tell you to eat bananas and drink orange juice, both excellent natural sources of potassium. If your potassium level stays low, your doctor may prescribe a potassium supplement or try a potassium-sparing drug instead. NEVER take salt or electrolyte supplements unless your doctor tells you to. Your doctor may prescribe a diuretic if you have high blood pressure or heart failure, sometimes in combination with other medications.

Vasodilators

The most common vasodilation drug is nitroglycerin, placed under your tongue to slowly dissolve. Vasodilators cause your arteries and veins to expand, making it easier for your heart to pump blood out and slowing the return flow of blood from your veins. This reduces your heart's workload, often easing attacks of ischemia (temporary insufficient oxygen to your heart muscle), which cause angina. Angina is the primary reason for prescribing some vasodilators. In addition to nitroglycerin, other common vasodilators are hydralazine, minoxidil, and reserpine.

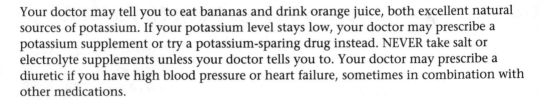

Take It to Heart

One man's side effect is another man's cure for baldness. The drug minoxidil, known better by its trade name Rogaine, sometimes increases hair growth—not an especially good thing when your back sprouts, but a panacea for male pattern baldness (though hair growth stops when you stop using the drug). Minoxidil now comes in a lotion form for hair growth that is available without a prescription.

Herbal and Naturopathic Remedies: Do They Work?

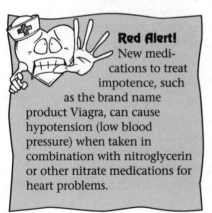

Red Alert!

New medications to treat impotence, such as the brand name product Viagra, can cause hypotension (low blood pressure) when taken in combination with nitroglycerin or other nitrate medications for heart problems.

Garlic, cayenne, and parsley sound more like the beginnings of a zesty marinara sauce than remedies to help lower blood pressure and blood cholesterol. Yet they've been popular "heart treatments" for centuries. Pectin—found in foods like apples, carrots, and grapefruit—binds with dietary fat, preventing its absorption into the body. Millions of people use herbal and nutritional supplements for a wide variety of health reasons, from chamomile for its calming effect to zinc for the reduction of cold symptoms.

Scientific evidence supporting the effectiveness of these approaches varies, in part because the remedies vary in potency and content. Government agencies don't monitor or regulate naturopathic production processes. Formulas differ among manufacturers. While many *herbal* and *naturopathic* remedies may be helpful, most are not scientifically proven.

Some herbal and naturopathic remedies can be harmful and even deadly, especially when used incorrectly or taken in combination with other remedies or drugs. Herbal remedies you take for other reasons can create unexpected problems, too.

Substances for weight loss and allergies often contain ephedra, an extract of the stimulant ephedrine. In products known variously as mahuang, desert tea, squaw tea, and whorehouse tea (a concoction once thought to cure syphilis and gonorrhea, which only antibiotics can do), ephedra raises blood pressure and pulse rate. If you have heart disease, ephedra stimulants can cause sudden death.

Also popular are preparations containing ginkgo, used to offset the unpleasant symptoms of menopause. Ginkgo appears to interfere with clotting, which is particularly hazardous if you're also taking an anticoagulant.

Another popular menopause remedy uses an herbcalled black cohosh, often taken in the form of a tea. In addition to affecting estrogen levels, black cohosh is a stimulant that can have vasodilation effects (causing your blood vessels to open).

The bottom line? In a word, *caution*. If herbal or natural remedies interest you, talk with your doctor about ways to integrate them safely into your life. The lack of scientific study and manufacturing inconsistencies make many doctors leery of these remedies; often, your doctor can't tell you what possible effects could result from combining them with each other or with prescribed medications, because no one knows. And sadly, there are disreputable products on the market that claim to cure everything from the common cold to cancer (and heart disease). They don't. For all its imperfections, modern medicine achieves impressive results. Don't forgo traditional treatment approaches in favor of unproven "cures." If something sounds too good to be true, it probably is.

The truth is, heart health requires your continual participation. You can't just take a pill—herbal or otherwise—and forget about your responsibility to your heart. You must

> **By Heart**
> *Naturopathic medicine*, or naturopathy, is a form of alternative medicine that uses substances found naturally in the environment for healing and to maintain health. Many such substances are *herbal*, derived from herbs found in the wild or cultivated for medicinal use. Conventional medicine is practiced by physicians who graduate from medical school and write "MD" after their names.

> **Red Alert!**
> Are you taking any herbal or naturopathic remedies for high blood pressure, high blood cholesterol levels, or any other reasons (even not heart-related)? Be sure to tell your doctor about them. Sometimes, naturopathic remedies and conventional medications can clash, producing unexpected effects. Bring in the bottles for your doctor to see.

balance your life using all that is available to you—diet, exercise, stress reduction techniques, and medical care—to keep your heart happy and healthy.

Chelation Therapy: Unsafe Plaque Eaters?

Chelation therapy for coronary artery disease sounds like a dream come true. You spend a couple hours each month with an IV (intravenous) solution running into your vein that dissolves accumulated fatty deposits from your arteries. And *voilà!* No more coronary artery disease.

Is it really this easy to get rid of those pesky arterial plaque deposits? Probably not. Doctors have long used chelation therapy to treat poisoning from heavy metals like lead and mercury. Chelates are substances that combine with these metals to convert them into less toxic materials that your body can then rapidly eliminate. Chelates occur naturally. They aid biochemical processes like *metabolism* (converting vitamins and minerals to energy that your body's cells can use) and allow your body to use medications like antibiotics.

Chelation therapy to reduce arterial plaque applies the same principle approach that draws heavy metals from the body. Arterial plaque contains a variety of minerals found naturally in the body (like iron, arsenic, and aluminum). The chelate—in this case, an amino acid called *ethylene diamine tetra acetic* acid (EDTA)—bonds with these minerals and draws them out of the plaque. In theory, the plaque begins to disintegrate over time as more and more of its building blocks disappear.

Most medical authorities, including the American Heart Association and the American College of Cardiology, view this use of chelation therapy as unproven. As yet, there's little scientific evidence to support claims of arterial cleansing, though there is some evidence that chelation therapy can result in kidney damage. Doctors worry that patients who might benefit from early intervention, such as balloon angioplasty, will delay in favor of chelation therapy. If you really want to help your body reduce arterial plaque, work through diet and exercise to lower your "bad" cholesterol to less than 100—research shows that arterial plaque begins to dissolve with very low LDL (low density lipoproteins) and VLDL (very low density lipoproteins) levels. We discuss "good" and "bad" cholesterol in detail in Chapter 14.

Procedures for Heart Health

Most medical procedures to restore heart health are invasive, which is to say they involve entering your body in some way. This, in turn, involves a certain level of risk. Be sure you understand what those risks are for you and what potential benefits the procedure offers. Discuss these matters with your doctor before you schedule any invasive procedures. Before you undergo an invasive procedure, your doctor will ask you to sign a statement of informed consent saying that you and your doctor have had this discussion, and you understand the procedure's possible risks and benefits.

Angioplasty: Unplugging Small Blockages

Angioplasty takes cardiac catheterization from diagnosis to treatment. Your doctor maneuvers a catheter through your arteries and into the blocked portion of a coronary artery. This catheter has a tiny balloon on the end that your doctor inflates by filling it with a saline solution using a syringe. This presses the blockage against the artery's walls. Often, your doctor will also insert a *stent*, or tiny coiled tube, into the area to keep the blockage from closing in again.

Angioplasty patients often go home in three or four days and are back to normal activities in two or three weeks. Your doctor may recommend angioplasty if you have just a single artery (at most, two arteries) blocked. When combined with a stent, angioplasty can provide long-lasting relief from arterial stenosis, or narrowing.

Coronary Artery Bypass: Constructing a Detour

Sometimes the only thing left to do for badly occluded, or blocked, coronary arteries is to surgically replace them. Surgeons may use a segment of vein from your leg or an artery from your chest wall (the mammary artery) to construct new coronary arteries. These grafts bypass the diseased arteries, rerouting the flow of blood.

By Heart
One of the most exciting developments of the 1990s was a spring-like coil called a *stent*. Often placed after balloon angioplasty or coronary bypass, a stent has tiny wires that hook it into the artery's wall. Within a few weeks, the artery's inner lining grows over the wires, leaving the stent inside the wall like a brace. Stents keep arteries from closing, prolonging the benefit of surgical interventions.

Take It to Heart
Coronary artery bypass grafts use arteries harvested from other parts of your body. The mammary artery in your chest is a popular choice because other arteries in those areas quickly expand to take over the circulation previously handled by the harvested artery.

Coronary artery bypass has become one of the most commonly performed surgeries in the United States, causing us to sometimes forget that it is open heart surgery. A machine called a heart–lung bypass machine takes over oxygenating your blood and "beats" for your heart, which doctors must stop to perform the surgery. Surgery takes between three and five hours and involves two or more surgeons (generally, one works on removing vein grafts from your leg while the other cuts through skin, muscle, and bone to expose your heart).

Most bypass patients spend a week or so in the hospital and six to eight weeks recovering at home. In the past, bypass operations sometimes had to be repeated after 10 years or so, as the new grafts eventually became clogged. New procedures that use stents to keep the grafts open may make repeat surgeries significantly less common.

Pacemakers: Going Steady

Early pacemakers were about the size of a transistor radio, if you remember that marvel of portability popular in the 1960s when the first pacemakers became available. Worn on the belt or on a strap over the shoulder, the early pacemaker used external wires to connect to a paddle-like electrode surgically placed in contact with the heart. The first internal, or implanted, pacemakers looked more like hockey pucks than emerging technology.

Cardio Care
Do you have a pacemaker? Avoid devices with strong electromagnetic fields, like older microwave ovens and high-voltage equipment, that can disrupt the signals your pacemaker sends to your heart. One source of potential danger is the security system at the airport. Tell security officers you have a pacemaker, and ask them to search you without using electronic or magnetic devices. Airports have special procedures for this.

Long-acting lithium batteries power today's electronic pacemakers. Microcircuitry makes these devices small enough to be unnoticeably implanted in a pocket of skin near the shoulder. A *fixed* pacemaker sends electrical impulses to your heart no matter what impulses your heart generates itself; a *demand* pacemaker sends tiny jolts only when your heart misses a beat or slows below a certain rate. A *dual-chamber* pacemaker can stimulate the atria as well as the ventricles to maintain synchronization. Most pacemakers implanted today are demand or dual-chamber; fixed pacemakers are rarely used.

It takes a minor surgical procedure, with only local anesthesia, to implant a pacemaker. After numbing the area, your doctor makes a small incision near your collarbone and inserts a catheter (tube) into the *subclavian vein* (a large vein under your collarbone). Your doctor then guides the pacemaker's leads (wires with electrodes at the tips) through the catheter and into your heart. A small pocket cut into the fleshy tissue of your chest holds the pacemaker's power supply. Having a pacemaker implanted may mean a day or two in the hospital, mostly so your doctor can monitor how your heart responds to its new partner.

Implantable Defibrillators: Shocks to Go

Some heart rhythm problems cause your ventricles to go into fibrillation (to flutter rapidly and uselessly). If not immediately corrected, ventricular fibrillation causes death. *Implantable cardioverter defibrillators* (ICDs) can send brief, regular impulses to your heart to thwart fibrillation, deliver a mild shock to redirect your heart back to a normal rhythm (called *cardioversion*), or give a stiff shock to jolt your heart out of a dangerous fibrillation.

Most people don't feel the first two actions, though defibrillation definitely packs a kick. Fainting during defibrillation is common and one of the risks of having an ICD.

Implanting an ICD is more complicated than implanting a pacemaker. After threading the ICD's leads into your heart, doctors must use the ICD to deliver a shock to be sure the unit works properly. Since this can be uncomfortable, most patients receive general anesthesia so they're asleep during the procedure. Recovery time is a day or two. Once implanted, an ICD's long-use batteries last about 7 years.

The same precautions for pacemakers apply to ICDs after implantation—avoid strong electromagnetic fields. If you have an ICD, your doctor will probably instruct you to call whenever it gives you a shock. Wear a medical alert necklace or bracelet saying that you have an ICD.

Radiofrequency Ablation: Energy Waves to Restore Rhythm

Certain kinds of tachycardia, particularly supraventricular tachyarrythmias, respond well to radiofrequency ablation. In this nonsurgical procedure, a cardiologist threads a thin catheter through your veins to the area of your heart where electrical impulses originate. An electrode at the tip of the catheter delivers a quick burst of radiofrequency energy that burns a very small number of heart muscle cells, causing them to die. This stops the cells from transmitting electrical impulses, restoring your heart to a regular rhythm. About 95 percent of people who undergo radiofrequency ablation leave the hospital with their arrythmias permanently cured. The procedure is often done on an outpatient basis.

Reversing Heart Problems Without Drugs or Surgery

For many years, common knowledge held that without intervention, coronary artery disease would worsen until it totally occluded the arteries, resulting in heart attack and death. This premise motivated extensive research to find safer, more effective ways to clear blockages through various surgical techniques.

Dean Ornish, M.D., took another approach. What if, he speculated, lifestyle changes alone could halt and even reverse coronary artery disease? To test his belief that they could, Dr. Ornish developed a rigorous regimen that combined a vegetarian diet with walking, meditation, stress-reducing activities, and group mental health therapy. He then enlisted volunteers with diagnosed coronary artery disease to participate in a study. In 82 percent, coronary blockages decreased and blood flow to the heart improved, measured by PET scans and computer-analyzed coronary angiograms. Of the fewer than half (47 percent) that improved in the control group, most implemented lifestyle changes on their own. While the experiment involved small numbers (41 people in the first study), the results are encouraging.

Take It to Heart

American physician Dean Ornish, M.D., began studying whether comprehensive, significant lifestyle changes could alter the course of heart disease in 1977. By 1990, he had clear evidence that it could, and published his findings. Since then, a number of medical centers across the United States have developed programs based on Ornish's strict regimen that integrates a low-fat, vegetarian diet; daily stress management techniques; and no smoking.

Is It Possible?

In his book, *Dr. Dean Ornish's Program for Reversing Heart Disease*, Ornish demands strict adherence to all of the program's elements, which include a vegetarian diet that is less than 10 percent fat. Ornish believes that, contrary to popular belief, it's sometimes easier to ask people to make major rather than moderate changes.

Red Alert! There is the possibility that a diet too low in fat can paradoxically decrease HDL (good cholesterol) and increase LDL (bad cholesterol). If you think the Ornish program might be right for you, ask your doctor first.

In an interview with journalist Bill Moyers for the PBS series *Healing and the Mind*, Ornish observes that healthcare professionals often make presumptions for people who, if they understood the benefits of major change, would choose that route.

"It's analogous to saying, 'We know you won't quit smoking, so we're not even going to tell you to try,'" Ornish told Moyers. "'Just smoke two packs a day instead of three.' What is true and what is easy are different issues."

Doctors need to tell patients what changes will make the most difference, Ornish believes, so they can make informed decisions. Those who really want to reverse their heart disease through radical change may think of it as choosing to enjoy, not limit, life.

Does It Really Work, and Can It Work for You?

For those willing to make the comprehensive changes that Ornish says are necessary to restore heart health and reverse heart disease, Ornish points to the results of his studies as evidence that his program can and does work. The change starts with finding motivation in joy rather than fear. Doctors have a patient's absolute attention in the first two weeks after a heart attack, Ornish points out, and then the fear wears off. In his program, Ornish tells Moyers, "We're not talking about how to live longer, or how to avoid a heart attack, but how to improve the quality and joy within your life, right now."

Are you willing to make a complete lifestyle change? If so, you, too, might overcome heart problems without surgery or drugs. But talk with your doctor before you start so that you'll understand how serious your heart disease is and what your options (and their consequences) are. Ornish's patients achieve results by strictly following his program and are under his (or another doctor's) supervision as they go through the program.

The Least You Need to Know

➤ Once disease takes hold of your heart, the most common interventions are drugs and procedures or surgery.

➤ Lifestyle changes are an element of any intervention; all treatment approaches work better when you also improve your diet, exercise regularly, and avoid smoking.

➤ If you want to use herbal or natural remedies as part of your treatment program, talk with your doctor. Some substances have harmful effects when heart disease exists or in combination with medications to treat heart problems.

➤ To get the most from your heart-healthy treatment program, take your medications properly. If you have trouble establishing a routine for taking your medications or experience side effects that you don't like, let your doctor know.

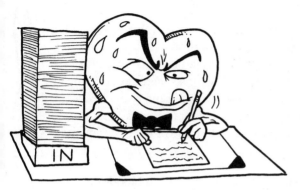

Chapter 8

When Your Pressure's Up

> **In This Chapter**
>
> ➤ Defining high blood pressure
>
> ➤ How to find out if you have high blood pressure
>
> ➤ Treatments for high blood pressure
>
> ➤ Special concerns for women

Everyone has blood pressure. Without it, your heart's work would be worthless—all that blood it pumps would go nowhere. And everyone's blood pressure goes up... and down. When your blood pressure goes up and stays up, it becomes a condition called *hypertension*. Doctors call hypertension "the silent killer" because you may not know you have it until it causes a heart attack or stroke. You can't feel it, hear it, or see it. Fifty million American adults—one in four—have hypertension; 40,000 of them die from it each year. High blood pressure is the leading cause of the 400,000 strokes that Americans suffer each year, and it is a significant risk factor for other heart disease. *Untreated* high blood pressure can shorten your life by 10 to 20 years.

Take It to Heart

British minister and scientist Stephen Hales (1677–1761) was the first to measure blood pressure. The year was 1733. A botanist by training and a physiologist by interest, Hales used a mercury-based gauge, adapted from one he developed to measure the pressure of sap in plants, to measure changes in the pressure of blood as it flows through the body. It was nearly 100 years before the stethoscope's development made practical today's method of listening to, rather than feeling, the pulse to take blood pressure measurements.

Hypertension can be primary—a disease condition of its own. High blood pressure also can be secondary, developing as the result of a disease condition elsewhere in your body. A prime example of high blood pressure as a secondary disease is hypertension resulting from kidney disease. Your kidneys do more than pass water from your body. They cleanse your blood of the biochemical wastes it collects on its rounds through your body, including salt compounds called *electrolytes* (potassium, sodium, magnesium, chloride, and phosphate, to name a few). When the levels of these salts in your blood are too high, they "suck" fluids from your body cells. Your kidneys then leave more water in your body to try to dilute the salts. The increased volume that results causes your blood pressure to go up. Heart failure affects electrolyte levels as well. And strokes can damage your brainstem, affecting its ability to regulate vital functions such as breathing.

The good news is worth dancing about, though. Hypertension is almost as preventable as it is dangerous. That's so important, we want to say it again so you can savor it as much as we do: Hypertension is almost as preventable as it is dangerous. (The most significant risk factor you *can't* influence is your family history; your gender and the presence of diabetes also affect your risk level.) If your blood pressure is normal now, five lifestyle factors can reduce your odds of getting hypertension to nearly zero:

➤ Maintaining a healthy weight

➤ Staying (or becoming) physically active

➤ Limiting your salt intake

➤ Drinking alcoholic beverages in moderation (no more than one or two drinks a day, if at all)

➤ Not smoking

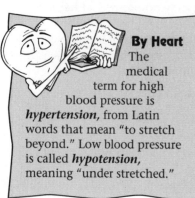

By Heart
The medical term for high blood pressure is *hypertension,* from Latin words that mean "to stretch beyond." Low blood pressure is called *hypotension,* meaning "under stretched."

That's all you have to do! Sounds simple, doesn't it? We know it's not. But in what other aspect of your life do you have such complete power to change the course of destiny? You truly have an opportunity to take your life in your hands!

What Is High Blood Pressure?

It's normal for your blood pressure to go up with exercise and stress. When it doesn't come back down, that's not normal. The simple definition of high blood pressure is diastolic or systolic readings that are above the normal range for a sustained time. Remember homeostasis, the body's ability to use its self-adjusting mechanisms to maintain a harmonious balance among its various systems? As your blood pressure rises, your body's systems adjust... for a while. So you don't see, hear, or feel anything different... for a while.

Has the thermostat in your house ever gone on the blink? Your furnace keeps running and your house heats up, but the thermostat still tells the furnace to pour it on. You feel OK for a while, then suddenly your house feels like an afternoon in August and you've run out of clothes to take off.

Your body's "thermostat" is your brainstem, which regulates base life functions—respiration, heart rate, blood pressure, and body temperature. With high blood pressure, your brainstem responds to signals from other organ systems (like your brain and nervous system) complaining that they're not getting enough blood. Sometimes these signals reflect a genuine inadequacy in blood supply. Accumulations of fatty deposits cause your arteries to narrow and stiffen, for example, reducing the amount of blood that can pass through them. In other circumstances, the signals are false, just little white lies. But your brainstem doesn't ask any questions—remember, this is not the seat of intelligence... it's the core of autonomous (automatic) function. Your body says "Crank it up!" and your brainstem says "You got it!" Your heart pumps harder, and for a while, your other body systems are happy—your body returns to a temporary state of homeostasis (albeit an unhealthy one).

But untreated high blood pressure is one of those vicious-cycle situations. The very increases your body systems demand worsen (or create) disease conditions that in turn increase the demands. More blood flowing at higher pressures through your arteries causes more fatty deposits, which cause your arteries to become more stiff, which reduces blood flow—and before you know it, those body systems are calling for more blood. While researchers know the damage primary hypertension can cause, they don't know exactly what causes it to develop in the first place.

How High Is Too High?

The higher your blood pressure goes, the greater your risk that you'll experience what we'll euphemistically call a catastrophic event. This could be a heart attack, a stroke, an aneurysm (a split in the wall of an artery allowing blood to escape), kidney disease, or even blindness. While the damage of these consequences is permanent, bringing your blood pressure under control (back to normal levels) can prevent these events from happening in the first place.

Normal blood pressure readings range from 90/60 to 140/90 (measured as millimeters of mercury, or mm/Hg). You have high blood pressure (hypertension) when *either number* is above the higher figures (140/90). Doctors classify high blood pressure into four stages, which they then assign to three risk groups. This process, called *risk stratification*, helps determine which treatment approaches are most appropriate.

Table 8.1 Stages of Hypertension

If Either Number of Your Blood Pressure Reading Is	You Have This Stage of Hypertension
130/85 to 139/89	High Normal
140/90 to 159/99	Stage 1
160/100 to 169/109	Stage 2
170/110 and higher	Stage 3

"White Coat" Hypertension

How do you feel when you're sitting in the exam room waiting for the doctor to come in? Your comfort level is probably proportionate to the amount of your own clothing that you still have on—there's something about those little paper gowns that ratchets up anxiety a few notches! If you've rushed from work, dashed from your car to the doctor's office, and raced to the bathroom before the nurse called your name, your body is physically stressed, too. Your body responds to the physical and emotional "fight or flight" crisis it senses by raising your blood pressure. When the nurse or doctor comes in to take a blood-pressure reading, yours is going to be high. If you feel especially anxious or revved up, let your doctor know. A repeat blood-pressure reading at the end of your visit often will show whether the first reading was falsely high.

Cardio Care

Does your list of favorite foods include bananas, cantaloupe, potatoes, red beans, or oranges? These high-potassium fruits and vegetables could help keep your blood pressure down. Research suggests a diet that includes moderate levels of potassium is helpful. Some medications for high blood pressure, especially diuretics, can draw potassium from your body. Don't take potassium supplements, though, unless you clear it with your doctor.

Can Blood Pressure Be Too Low?

What about low blood pressure, or *hypotension*? Some people have blood pressure readings lower than normal that don't affect them at all. Sometimes hypotension does cause problems. Unlike hypertension (with its lack of symptoms its most dangerous feature), hypotension makes its presence known primarily by causing dizziness and fainting—not enough blood gets to the brain, so the brain starts to shut down nonessential functions such as consciousness. These symptoms are pretty hard to ignore, so people who experience them usually see a doctor right away.

You don't hear as much about hypotension because it's not nearly as common as hypertension. Hypotension is usually a consequence of another condition (diabetes, shock) or a medication (for example, some antidepressants and sometimes drugs given to treat hypertension). Treatment involves identifying and correcting the underlying problem.

Getting a Reading

Taking a blood pressure reading is fairly simple to do; often, a nurse or medical technician will take the reading before your doctor sees you. If you feel overly anxious or you've just raced from your car to the office to avoid being late for your appointment, ask to wait a few minutes until you calm down. Did you have a cup of coffee, a cola drink, or a cigarette within an hour of your doctor's visit? Caffeine and nicotine, drugs these products contain, raise blood pressure. If your doctor suspects high blood pressure (you have a higher than normal reading or several risk factors), he or she may take several readings—in both arms, while you're sitting, and while you're lying down.

Sphygmomanometer: Off the Cuff

The most accurate sphygmomanometer remains the mercury column that hangs on the wall in your doctor's office. There's very little that can go wrong with this model, unlike electronic and gauge models that need regular calibration. If the blood pressure cuff is too small for your arm, it doesn't completely stop the circulation and give a possibly inaccurate reading. Some doctors' offices use a blood pressure cuff that has a dial gauge attached.

Monitoring Your Blood Pressure at Home

A number of companies market home blood pressure monitoring kits. Some are easier to use and more reliable than others. If your doctor wants you to monitor your blood pressure at home, ask for recommendations about what to buy. A pharmacist can also offer suggestions and may allow you to try out different models to see which one works best for you.

When taking your own blood pressure (or having a family member help you), be sure to sit comfortably for a few minutes first so you're calm when you take the reading. Check your blood pressure at the same time each day.

And even if you monitor your blood pressure at home, be sure to visit your doctor as recommended. This gives you a chance to compare your readings to the one your doctor gets and to discuss any concerns about your blood pressure. Your doctor also uses your visit to check other aspects of your health, which is especially important with a condition like hypertension that can affect other body systems.

How Do You Know When You've Got It?

Ah, the $64,000 question! Unless you know what your blood pressure reading is, you *don't* know when you have high blood pressure. This potentially deadly condition has few warning signs. Most doctors' visits start with a blood pressure check for this reason. Many health departments, fire departments, and public clinics offer free blood pressure screening. Some employers and schools schedule onsite blood-pressure testing and health fairs.

Who's at Risk for Hypertension?

Many of the same risk factors for heart disease in general apply to hypertension—family history, diet, inactivity, obesity, diabetes, and smoking, to name a few. Your risk of high blood pressure, regardless of any other risk factors, increases as you grow older. About 20 percent of Americans who are under the age of 50 have high blood pressure. The percentage more than doubles for the next decade of life, and by age 60, more people than not have high blood pressure.

Just for YOU
For reasons researchers don't fully understand, African-Americans are twice as likely to develop hypertension. The probabilities go up with each additional risk factor, especially diabetes and obesity. African-Americans who have hypertension are likely to have it more severely, too.

Do you weigh a bit more than you should? (Up to 40 percent of Americans do.) Research shows a connection between extra weight and increased blood pressure. Excess body fat affects the ability of capillaries to dilate (relax), which in turn affects the force of your heart's contractions. The other aspect of obesity that influences blood pressure is lack of exercise.

And as important as the risk factors for high blood pressure are, remember that high blood pressure is itself a risk factor for other kinds of heart disease. Doctors classify your risk level according to the number of risk factors you have. They call these classifications *risk groups*.

Table 8.2   Risk Groups

If You Have	Then You're
➤ No risk factors, and ➤ No target organ disease, and ➤ No known heart disease	Risk Group A
➤ At least one risk factor (not diabetes), and ➤ No target organ disease, and ➤ No known heart disease	Risk Group B
➤ Target organ disease, and/or ➤ Known heart disease, and/or ➤ Diabetes	Risk Group C

How Do Doctors Figure It Out?

Diagnosing hypertension is not quite as simple as taking a blood pressure reading. First of all, there are a number of circumstances (like activity and anxiety) that can raise your blood pressure temporarily, even though most of the time, your readings are normal.

If your blood pressure reading is high, your doctor will probably recheck it over a few weeks to a few months to see if your readings are consistently high. Your doctor will also ask questions about your family history and any health problems you've had (remember your genogram!). Doctors also look for *target organ damage*—injury to organs like your eyes, heart, and kidneys—and check for other conditions that can cause secondary hypertension, like thyroid disease. Your doctor may order additional heart tests (like an ECG, echocardiogram, or exercise tolerance ECG) if you seem to have such damage, though these tests aren't necessary to diagnose hypertension.

What Women Need to Know

Hormones protect women against high blood pressure as they do other heart diseases. Hypertension is more likely in men between the ages of 35 and 64 than it is in women of the same age range. As the estrogen buffer fades, however, the balance shifts. After age 65, women are more likely than men to develop the condition. And speaking of hormones, do you take birth control pills? In some women, this popular form of contraception raises blood pressure.

Several lifestyle changes that reduce your chance of high blood pressure and heart disease may also lower your risk for osteoporosis, an often debilitating drain of calcium from your bones after menopause. Exercise helps bones retain calcium, and it appears that cutting back on the amount of salt in your diet lowers the level of calcium your kidneys excrete.

> **Cardio Care**
> New studies show that many people (especially older Americans) can lower high blood pressure enough to stop taking medication by losing some weight and decreasing their salt intake. If you have high blood pressure, ask your doctor if these lifestyle changes could help you.

Getting It Under Control

Hypertension is most dangerous when untreated. Once you develop high blood pressure, it won't get better without some help from you. If your blood pressure is in the high-normal range (no higher than 139/89), your doctor will probably recommend lifestyle changes to bring it under control. Diet and exercise have the added benefit of weight loss; all three influence blood pressure. If lifestyle changes bring your blood pressure to a normal level and keep it there, you won't need medication.

Your risk-group classification helps your doctor determine what course of treatment to take for stages 1, 2, and 3 hypertension (see tables 8.1 through 8.3). Once you start taking medication to control your blood pressure, you'll need to take it for the rest of your life, even after your blood pressure returns to normal. Remember, these are general guidelines. Your personal circumstances and your doctor's judgment determine what treatment approach is most appropriate for you.

Take It to Heart

Today, nearly all primary hypertension (high blood pressure not caused by another disease) is treatable with medication. Twenty-five years ago, this wasn't the case. Hypertension that doctors couldn't treat was considered malignant—it would progress until it had fatal consequences, as it did for President Franklin D. Roosevelt (in the form of a cerebral hemorrhage). A new class of drugs developed in the 1970s, called beta blockers, finally conquered even stubborn primary high blood pressure. Much of the damage untreated hypertension causes is permanent, however.

Table 8.3   Risk Levels and Treatment Approaches

If Your Stage Is	And Your Risk Group Is	Your Likely Treatment Is*
High-Normal	Group A	Lifestyle changes, check in 1 year
	Group B	Lifestyle changes, check in 6 months to 1 year
	Group C	Lifestyle changes + medication, check in 2 months and yearly
Stage 1	Group A	Lifestyle changes, check in 1 year
	Group B	Lifestyle changes, check in 6 months
	Group C	Lifestyle changes + medication, check in 2 months and yearly
Stage 2	Any	Lifestyle changes + medication, check in 1 month and every 6 months
Stage 3	Any	Lifestyle changes + medication, check in 1 week, 1 month, and every 6 months

These are general guidelines. Your doctor will recommend treatment for you that considers your personal circumstances.

Lifestyle, Lifestyle, Lifestyle

We get to say it again: You can prevent nearly all hypertension by making heart-healthy lifestyle choices that reduce, eliminate, and even reverse hypertension risk factors. Lifestyle changes control about 25 percent of all diagnosed hypertension. Here are some of the choices you can make:

➤ **Pass on the salt.** Most Americans consume far more salt than the body needs—up to 20 times more. Too much salt draws additional fluid from your body into your bloodstream, increasing the volume of blood and the amount of work your heart must do to move it through your circulatory system. Limit the salt you add to your food to about a teaspoonful a day, and avoid foods that are high in sodium (bacon, fast foods, canned goods, and soy sauce are common examples).

➤ **Drop the fat.** High levels of dietary fat contribute to atherosclerosis and arteriosclerosis, two conditions often present in high blood pressure and other heart disease. Less fat in your diet means less fat floating through your arteries.

➤ **Fitness is health.** We're talking lung power here, not abs of steel. Just walking at a brisk pace for 30 to 45 minutes at a time gives your body a decent aerobic workout, strengthening your arteries and heart as well as your legs.

➤ **Moderation.** A little(up to three ounces of alcohol) benefits your heart, alcohol consumption comes with its own set of health risks. If you don't drink now, don't start.

➤ **Temper, temper.** Anger and stress make the blood pressure rise, sometimes suddenly and drastically. Several studies connect a stressful lifestyle with elevated blood pressure. Stress also can trigger *ischemia* (temporary shortage of blood to your heart muscle).

➤ **Don't smoke.** Nicotine, the main drug in tobacco, elevates blood pressure directly. Cigarette smoking compounds most risk factors for heart disease.

Red Alert!
While a drink or two a day might be good for your heart, too much is dangerous. More than three drinks a day have a direct toxic effect on your heart. Binge drinking (consuming large amounts of alcohol infrequently, such as on weekends) puts you at risk for atrial fibrillation.

When Is Drug Therapy Necessary?

If lifestyle changes fail to bring your blood pressure back to a normal level in five to six weeks, your doctor will prescribe a medication that will. These medications fall into several categories, or classes; your doctor will try to match your situation with the medication most likely to bring your blood pressure under control.

Cardio Care

Do you take your medication as the instructions on the label tell you to? Nearly half of all people do not, with sometimes serious consequences. It's particularly important to take your medication at about the same time each day to keep a constant level of the drug in your body. Try taking your pills with other regular activities, like meals.

Medications prescribed for high blood pressure sometimes deliver undesirable side effects along with their pressure-reducing actions. Doctors and pharmacists have no way of knowing in advance if you are likely to have side effects from a particular medication. Ask what side effects to watch for, and let your doctor know immediately if you experience any of them. For most people with hypertension, there are a number of medications to choose from, and finding the one that works for you is a process of trial and error.

Whatever you do, DON'T stop taking blood pressure medication because you don't like its side effects! Instead, talk with your doctor, who might adjust your dose or switch you to another medication. Once you start taking medication for high blood pressure, you'll need to do so for the rest of your life. It's especially hazardous to stop blood pressure medication suddenly, because your blood pressure may skyrocket.

Table 8.4 Common Antihypertensive Drugs

Drug	Action	Reason Prescribed/Comments
ACE inhibitors	Stop kidneys from converting renin to angiotensin II, chemicals that cause capillaries to constrict	Not as effective in African-Americans; often drug of choice if kidney disease, diabetes, or heart failure is also present; expensive
Alpha blockers	Block signals that cause capillaries to constrict	Often in combination with meds; can cause blood pressure to drop suddenly upon standing
Beta blockers	Reduce the rate and force of the heart's pumping action by acting on the autonomic nervous system	Often the first drug tried; sometimes in combination with diuretics; also used to relieve angina (and migraine)
Calcium channel blockers	Slow movement of calcium across membranes of heart-muscle cells to slow their contraction	Usually third in blockers line of choices; cost $500 to $800 a year; may be combined with other antihypertensives
Diuretics ("water pills")	Increase sodium and water excretion by the kidneys, which decreases fluid in the blood vessels	Reduce blood volume; often prescribed with other blood pressure medication; very inexpensive (about $10 a year)

The Least You Need to Know

➤ High blood pressure often shows no symptoms.

➤ Undetected and untreated hypertension can lead to strokes, heart attacks, kidney damage, and damage to the blood vessels in the back of the eye (hypertensive retinopathy).

➤ Changes in diet and increased exercise are the most effective lifestyle changes you can make to prevent and sometimes reverse high blood pressure.

➤ Once you start taking medication to control high blood pressure, you'll need to take it always. Take your medication as the label instructs, and never stop without talking to your doctor.

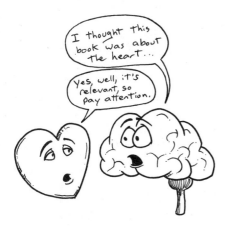

Chapter 9

Stroke: Brain Attack

In This Chapter

➤ The devastating legacy of stroke

➤ Determining your risk of stroke: A self-quiz

➤ Diagnosis and treatment

➤ Who's at special risk?

What do you think of when you hear the word "stroke?" Do you think *end of the road*? About one-third of all strokes are fatal, claiming 140,000 lives a year in the United States. Do you think *debilitating*? Stroke is the leading cause of adult disability. About half of those who survive a stroke need some level of help with daily living activities; 10 percent require long-term institutional care. Do you think *can't happen to me*? Take a look at your watch or a clock with a second hand. Count off 53 seconds. Another person suffers a stroke. What keeps you from being next?

The best cure for stroke is prevention. Researchers say that new therapies combined with lifestyle changes to reduce controllable risks have the potential to prevent 80 percent of all strokes. Early intervention is the next best thing. Thanks to new technologies and aggressive intervention (mostly early diagnosis and treatment of hypertension), the death rate from stroke dropped more than two-thirds between 1950 and 1993.

The Heart Disease Connection

Here you are, reading a book about your heart, and all of a sudden, we've jumped to your brain. What does a stroke have to do with heart disease? More than you think, as it turns out. Even though we call a stroke a "brain attack" and its symptoms are neurological, stroke belongs to the cardiovascular (heart and blood vessel) family of diseases. All the heart disease risk factors apply. In fact, certain heart problems (like high blood pressure and heart attacks) increase your risk of stroke.

Strokes result from one of two circumstances: Not enough blood (blockage) or too much blood (hemorrhage) reaching a portion of your brain. One of three events causes *ischemic*, or blockage, strokes, which account for 80 percent of all strokes:

➤ A blood clot forms in your artery (thrombosis).

➤ A blood clot or piece of arterial plaque breaks free and moves through your arteries until it gets stuck (embolism).

➤ An artery becomes extremely narrow, restricting blood flow (stenosis).

Hemorrhagic strokes are far less common and often result from an aneurysm, or weakened artery wall that ruptures. Aneurysms can be *congenital* (present from birth) or the consequence of *atherosclerosis* (the buildup of fatty materials in the arteries).

Whatever the cause, a stroke damages brain tissue. How this affects you depends on where and how extensive the damage is. In general, damage to the right side of your brain affects the left side of your body and vice versa. Damage to the left side of your brain can also affect your speech, since in most people, the speech center is located in the left brain.

For such a small organ (less than 2 percent of your bodyweight), your brain has an enormous appetite. It consumes 25 percent of your body's oxygen and nearly 70 percent of its glucose (sugar). There's no grace period when a stroke deprives brain tissue of these vital nutrients—damage is immediate and permanent, and it gets worse the longer the starvation continues.

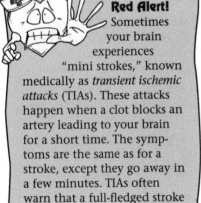

By Heart
There are two broad kinds of stroke: *ischemic* and *hemorrhagic*. Ischemic means "to block"; ischemic strokes result from a blockage in the artery and account for about 80 percent of all strokes. Hemorrhagic means "to bleed"; hemorrhagic strokes occur when an artery leaks or ruptures, spilling blood into the brain or the space surrounding it.

Red Alert!
Sometimes your brain experiences "mini strokes," known medically as *transient ischemic attacks* (TIAs). These attacks happen when a clot blocks an artery leading to your brain for a short time. The symptoms are the same as for a stroke, except they go away in a few minutes. TIAs often warn that a full-fledged stroke is on the way.

Hypertension: Pressure Cooker

Hypertension, or high blood pressure, is the number-one cause of stroke. Have you ever placed your thumb over the business end of a garden hose (or attached a spray nozzle) to increase the pressure of the water spraying out, then had the hose spring a leak? Hypertension can have a similar effect on your arteries, causing a weakened wall to split. And all that blood rushing through can dislodge bits of arterial plaque, sending them swirling through your system.

If you have high blood pressure or other risk factors for stroke, your doctor listens to the arteries in your neck (carotids) with a stethoscope. Plaque accumulations in these arteries are an early indication that you could be headed for a stroke. Sometimes your doctor can hear characteristic sounds called *bruits* that signal an increase in turbulence as your blood flows over the plaque.

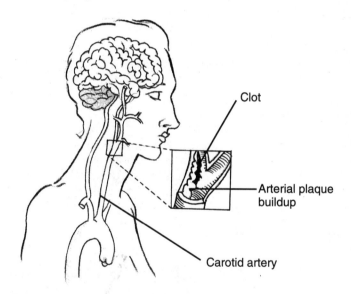

Clot

Arterial plaque buildup

Carotid artery

Plaque that builds up in your arteries can eventually plug the artery, preventing blood from flowing through.

After a Heart Attack

Have you had a heart attack? Then sit up and pay attention, because your risk of stroke is even higher. During a heart attack, your heart may stop pumping blood completely. This leaves your body—and your oxygen-hungry brain—without the blood supply that brings fresh oxygen. This can cause stroke-like damage in parts of the brain. And remember that most heart attacks result from blocked coronary arteries. These blockages can release tiny particles of arterial plaque, or even blood clots, into your bloodstream. If you have blocked arteries in your heart, chances are you have them elsewhere in your body, too. Conversely, if you've had a stroke, your risk of heart attack is much greater. This shouldn't come as a surprise, since the same circumstances can cause either condition.

> **Take It to Heart**
>
> Old ideas, like old habits, die hard. Once there was little hope for stroke victims. While recent innovations in stroke diagnosis and treatment have upended traditional thinking about the outlook for stroke patients, their absorption into common practice takes time to ripple through the medical community. Research using new drugs and sophisticated technology takes place at major medical centers in large cities. About 50 major medical centers throughout the country have formed *Acute Stroke Teams* (ASTs) to help spread the expertise. ASTs assist small hospitals to develop procedures that approach stroke as a treatable medical emergency rather than an inevitable debilitation.

The High Cost of Hesitation

The difference between walking out of the hospital in a week or less following a stroke and spending weeks or months in a rehabilitation center is often three hours or less if you have an ischemic stroke. Doctors can now administer new and powerful clot-dissolving drugs that can literally reverse a stroke. The catch is that this treatment is only effective if it takes place within three hours of your stroke. Get to the hospital emergency room right away if you think you could be having a stroke. Don't waste time worrying about whether it's "just nothing," especially if you know you have some risk factors. Prompt diagnosis and treatment can make sure "nothing" is precisely what your experience ends up being!

> **Red Alert!**
> Clot busters can save you from death or permanent damage from a stroke—but only if you get them in time. *These drugs must be given within three hours of when your stroke starts.* Don't wait to see if you're really having a stroke before you go to the emergency room. You can't tell anyway—even doctors need sophisticated tests to confirm a stroke.

High-Tech Tests: Fast-Track Diagnosis

If your symptoms suggest a stroke, emergency room doctors are likely to whisk you off for a CT (computerized tomography) scan. This sophisticated diagnostic tool tells doctors not so much whether you're having a stroke (as it's happening, a stroke is almost impossible to detect) as whether other conditions exist that could cause your symptoms (like a tumor or abscess). A CT scan also shows hemorrhaging in the brain, helping doctors determine what kind of stroke you're having. This is critical because treatments for an ischemic stroke (thrombolytics and anticoagulants) will worsen a hemorrhagic stroke by making it bleed even more. Followup tests to determine what caused your stroke might include any of the procedures described in Chapter 6, "Straight to the Heart," that are used to assess heart disease.

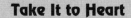

Take It to Heart

The University of California-Los Angeles (UCLA) developed a three-minute test to help paramedics determine whether someone is having a stroke. After ruling out seizures and similar disorders, paramedics instruct the person to perform simple motor skill exercises, like smiling and lifting each arm. Paramedics repeat the test several times and note any changes. Doctors hope widespread use of the test will get treatment started more quickly.

TPA and Streptokinase: Clot Busters

Who you gonna call when you've got a nasty clot? Clot busters! The most exciting innovation in stroke (and heart attack) treatment in the past decade is the development of drugs technically known as *thrombolytics*. When given intravenously (through a needle into your vein), thrombolytics rapidly dissolve clots, "unplugging" blocked arteries to restore blood flow. The most common of these drugs are streptokinase and *tissue plasminogen activator* (TPA).

You must receive these drugs within three hours of the onset of your stroke for them to be effective. TPA and streptokinase are very expensive (more than $2,000 a dose). Providers and insurers agree that this is a small price to pay when it saves 10 times that amount in hospital costs—not to mention the priceless value of saving a life.

Cardio Care
If you need further incentive to end alcohol use, consider this. Chronic alcohol use often causes microscopic bleeding in the intestines and other organs, and interferes with your body's blood-clotting mechanisms. This raises your risk of stroke. Yet giving you clot busters to stop your stroke could cause you to bleed to death.

Keeping the Lid on High Blood Pressure

A stroke sends your body's homeostasis into a tailspin. When your brain loses its blood supply, it sends frantic messages to your heart to get things back to normal *now*. Unfortunately, these messages are like the *Titanic's* captain telling the engine room to crank up the boilers—it doesn't fix the problem. But your heart dutifully responds, and your blood pressure skyrockets.

It takes from a few days to a few weeks for your body to restore its equilibrium, during which time your doctor may use intravenous antihypertensive drugs to gradually lower your blood pressure. This is a delicate balancing act itself, however, because your body may not respond in the expected ways while it's under the influence of your stroke. Since your blood pressure will slowly return to normal, the hospital staff will monitor your readings and adjust your medication to keep pace.

Know the Signs

Strokes don't often offer many clues that they are about to happen. They do provide clear signs that they are underway, however, and you should know what they are.

Warning Signs of Stroke

➤ Sudden weakness in your hand, arm, or leg

➤ Numbness on one side of your face or body

➤ Sudden inability to see out of one eye

➤ Sudden inability to understand what others are saying, or difficulty speaking

➤ Sudden dizziness or loss of balance

➤ Sudden, severe headache

What's Your Risk?: A Self-Quiz

The risks for stroke are much the same as those for heart disease in general. These factors are particularly relevant for stroke.

	Yes	No
Are you a woman over age 35 who smokes and takes birth control pills?	_____	_____
Do you have high blood pressure?	_____	_____
Are you African-American?	_____	_____
Have other family members had strokes?	_____	_____
Do you have two or more risk factors for heart disease?	_____	_____
Are you over age 65?	_____	_____
Do you smoke?	_____	_____

Every "yes" response increases your risk for stroke. If you have three or more "yes" responses, make an appointment with your doctor for a checkup, and discuss what you can do to lower your risk.

Who's at Risk?

What's your stroke-risk score? Even if it's low, don't feel you can just plop your laurels on the couch. Stroke can strike anyone at any time. If you're at risk for any other kind of heart disease, you're at risk for stroke. If you've been diagnosed with atrial fibrillation, you're also at risk for stroke and probably already take medication to regulate your heart's rhythm. Atrial fibrillation can cause blood to pool in your heart, which increases the chance for clots to form.

African-Americans

Researchers aren't certain why stroke rates for African-Americans are twice those Caucasian-Americans. African-Americans also are more likely to have less treatable hemorrhagic strokes. It seems to be a situation where "the whole is greater than the sum of its parts."

Health researchers believe an interaction of multiple risk factors is at the bottom of these statistics. Certain combinations seem to be more potent, like diabetes and high blood pressure together. African-Americans also face a risk three times that of other ethnic groups for hypertension, which is a primary cause of stroke.

Some of these risk factors are controllable, like smoking (in 1996, an estimated 32 percent of African-American men and 24 percent of African-American women smoked cigarettes). Physical inactivity, obesity, and diabetes are also key risk factors, just as they are for other heart diseases. So what do you do about these numbers if you're an African-American? You can't change your heritage or your family history. But you can change other factors. Stay on those controllable risks—eat right, exercise regularly, don't smoke, and have your blood pressure checked every six to twelve months.

Cardio Care
If you know you have risk factors for stroke, ask your doctor about aspirin therapy. Aspirin is a mild anticoagulant that seems to help prevent clots from forming. The typical dose is one baby aspirin or one-half adult aspirin daily. Don't start taking aspirin without talking to your doctor, though. If your risk is higher for hemorrhagic strokes, you don't want to take anything that could cause bleeding.

What Women Need to Know

Women face a greater risk of stroke than men do when other risk factors are present. Women who smoke, have diabetes, have high blood pressure, are overweight, and don't exercise are courting stroke. More women than men who have strokes die from them or have subsequent heart attacks. Women over age 35 who take birth-control pills and also smoke are playing with fire in more ways than one; this combination puts them at a particularly high risk. Do bleeding (hemorrhagic) strokes run in your family? These strokes seem to strike women at an earlier age and more frequently than men.

Over 55

Ah, here we go again with the aging. It's sad but true—the older you are, the higher your risk for stroke. About 28 percent of strokes happen in people under the age of 55. After that, your risk doubles for each decade that passes. Though you can't stop aging (not yet, anyway!), you can minimize other risk factors that are within your control.

Smokers Beware

Nicotine, the main chemical ingredient in tobacco, raises your blood pressure as soon as it migrates from your lungs to your bloodstream. (If you chew, it's absorbed through the capillaries that nourish the mucous membranes inside your mouth.) High blood pressure, remember, is the major cause of strokes. Smoking also accelerates atherosclerosis and compounds other risk factors for heart disease.

Red Alert! Don't take aspirin if you're already taking a "blood thinner" like warfarin, unless your doctor tells you to. Doing so greatly increases your risk of uncontrollable bleeding (hemorrhage), since both drugs affect clotting.

Life After a Stroke

Your life after a stroke could be about what it was before, especially if you got prompt treatment that prevented or reversed any damage. Early and aggressive physical and speech therapy helps those who do have permanent damage, such as partial paralysis and speech problems, relearn lost skills. Ongoing treatment for many stroke survivors includes high blood pressure medication and anticoagulants like warfarin or aspirin.

The Least You Need to Know

➤ Seek prompt medical attention for symptoms of stroke. "Clot buster" drugs only work within three hours of the stroke's onset.

➤ Age is the most important *uncontrollable* risk factor and smoking and hypertension are the most important *controllable* risk factors for stroke.

➤ An aspirin a day can reduce your risk of stroke by preventing blood clots from forming. Ask your doctor before you start taking aspirin, because aspirin therapy isn't for everyone (especially people already taking anticoagulants).

➤ Early, aggressive physical and speech therapy can help you return to a productive life even if your stroke leaves you with permanent damage.

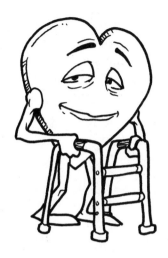

Heart Healing

There's nothing like a heart attack to put you in touch with the frailty of life. Indeed, when today's baby boomers wailed their first cries, a heart attack was a death sentence. More people died than not. Even if your heart attack didn't end your life, it ended life as you knew it. Survivors lived either as cardiac cripples, unable to engage in physical activity, or in fearful caution that any exertion would result in complete debilitation. This perception started to change in the 1950s when President Dwight D. Eisenhower suffered a major heart attack while in office. His doctors, spurred by recent developments in treating heart disease, encouraged him to return to the activities he loved—the presidency, golfing, and playing with his grandchildren.

Today, about two-thirds of those who have heart attacks survive. With appropriate treatment, they return to productive lives. That treatment can range from a few nights in the hospital and medication to angioplasty or bypass surgery—followed, of course, by life-long heart-healthy lifestyle changes.

Do You Know the Code? A Quick (Fun) Quiz

"So, didja have a pizza or a cabbage?" Feel like you've dropped down the rabbit hole right behind Alice? The medical wonderland has a language of its own, and unless you "know the code," you'll be hopelessly lost. Test your translation skills on these! Mark the answer that defines the word or phrase.

Pizza

_____ Gourmet food for couch potatoes

_____ All five food groups in a single meal

_____ Percutaneous transluminal coronary angioplasty

Cabbage

_____ Holding area for babies before they're born

_____ Odd-looking dolls

_____ Coronary artery bypass graft

Ball-and-cage

_____ Early sign of spring training

_____ Kinder, gentler variation on ball-and-chain

_____ Artificial heart valve with a ball that moves back and forth inside a thin wire cage to block or allow blood flow

Pig heart

_____ Someone who eats too much

_____ Someone who, in his or her heart of hearts, isn't really a very nice person

_____ Heart valve from a pig, transplanted to replace a diseased valve in a human heart

Cad

_____ Less than gentlemanly

_____ Youngster who carries golf bags

_____ Coronary artery disease

I See You

____ Your gown's open in the back

____ Child playing peek-a-boo

____ Intensive care unit

If you marked the last choice for each, you're a lingo star! (For extra credit, use them all in one sentence.)

Open Up: Balloon Angioplasty to the Rescue

So you had just a little problem, relatively speaking, a single blockage that started your heart complaining. Balloon angioplasty, more formally known as *percutaneous transluminal coronary angioplasty* (PCTA), takes care of that in less than an hour. Before you know it, you're back in your hospital bed, your heart beating easy with its renewed blood supply. You'll probably stay three or four days, just to be sure everything's OK. After you go home, rest and relax for two or three weeks. Though you only have a small incision where the catheter entered your vein to show for your experience, your body has nonetheless been through a traumatic time. Your doctor may refer you to a cardiac rehabilitation program to set up an exercise plan and learn how to change your cooking and eating habits.

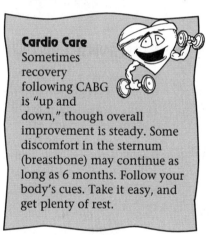

Cardio Care
Sometimes recovery following CABG is "up and down," though overall improvement is steady. Some discomfort in the sternum (breastbone) may continue as long as 6 months. Follow your body's cues. Take it easy, and get plenty of rest.

CABG: So You've Joined the "Big Zipper" Club!

Coronary arteries moving blood about like the expressway moves traffic at rush hour? *Coronary artery bypass graft* (CABG) surgery gives you a whole new set. When you first wake up after surgery, you may feel more like part of the high-tech machinery that surrounds you than the human race. Little happens with your body that escapes monitoring. But in just a few days, most of the equipment is gone, and you're actually left alone for longer than five minutes at a time. You dangle your feet from the side of your bed for a while, then decide you just have to see it. You manage to totter to the mirror over the sink, and there it is. Though it looks like it stretches from your chin to your belly button, your incision is really only about six inches long. All that orange stuff painted on your chest is the antiseptic solution used to clean your skin before surgery. And yes, those are staples holding your incision closed—as odd as that seems, staples are less uncomfortable, easier to remove, and leave less of a scar than stitches. They come out about five days after surgery. (The wires that hold your sternum together while it heals are yours for keeps.) You're officially a member of the "Big Zipper" club!

Take It to Heart

Anesthesia is a wonderful thing. It makes it possible for you to sleep so deeply doctors can open your chest and repair your heart, and you don't feel a thing (until you wake up, of course). But anesthesia leaves some effects behind that you'll have to tend to when you wake up. The gases used for anesthesia irritate your lungs a bit, and your lungs try to soothe themselves by producing more fluid. Coughing and deep breathing, even though they hurt, help prevent pneumonia. Sitting and standing keep the fluids from pooling at the bottom of your lungs.

Dealing with Post-Operative Pain

Don't worry, that train won't stay parked on your chest for long. The first day or so after surgery, you might even feel like it's using that nifty six-inch incision running down the center of your chest for its track. For about a week, the "pain train" will make pretty regular runs along that track. With all that coughing and deep breathing they make you do, it's little wonder you hurt! And what's with those nurses who come 'round to rouse you from a sound sleep to walk, *walk* of all things when you can't even turn over in bed without help? But excruciating as this all feels at first, your innards won't come ripping out, and even your unsteady shuffles to the hallway and back work wonders for your recovery.

Cardio Care

It's common to think you should wait until you hurt before you take a pain pill. It's also a mistake. It takes time—45 minutes to 2 hours—for pain medication to reach a high enough concentration in your blood to give you relief. By taking pain medication regularly for the first 10 to 14 days after heart surgery, you keep your relief level fairly constant—and yourself comfortable.

Believe it or not, by the time you leave for home less than two weeks later, you'll be turning, coughing, walking, and more, mostly without much pain or help. No little white lies from us—we'll tell you right up front that those sneezes are going to get you for a while yet. But even this, too, shall pass.

Your hospital gown is *not* a martyr's robe (how stoic can you be, anyway, with your back half shining at so many complete strangers?). Heart surgery hurts and everyone knows it, so there's no reason for you to act like yours doesn't. After all, someone has just sliced your chest muscles, sawed through your breastbone, and reconstructed part of your heart. Pain is natural and normal. Like the pain of childbirth, your pain after heart surgery has a purpose. It, too, gives new life—this time, to you.

For the first 24 to 36 hours after surgery, you'll get pain medication right in your IV (intravenous solution running fluids and nutrients into your vein). After you move from the intensive or cardiac care unit to a regular hospital room, you'll switch to oral pain pills. Take them. Suffering doesn't make you stronger or braver. Pain makes you want to lay very still, and that's about the worst thing you can do. So take your pain pills when it's time to take them, *before* the pain becomes unbearable. You won't get addicted for the short time you'll be on them, though you will feel more comfortable and interested in moving your recovery forward.

Should I Be Going Home So Soon?

Last week you roared to the hospital in an ambulance, breathing thanks only to the kindness of strangers. Today, you're leaving in a wheelchair (hospital policy) as a card-carrying, scar-bearing member of the zipper club. You're thankful to be alive... but is it really OK to be going home so soon after coming so close to losing your life? In a word, yep. Indeed, 15 or 20 years ago, it was common to stay in the hospital for two, three, even four weeks following open heart surgery. But practice perfects procedure.

Surgeons replace the coronary arteries of more than half a million Americans every year. And even though you may feel more secure in the hospital (in case something goes wrong), study after study shows you'll recover much more quickly in the comfort of your own home. Any unexpected events are most likely to happen in the first 48 hours.

How Long Does It Take to Feel Better?

You'll still be pretty sore when you leave the hospital, and you may find just the drive home wears you out. This is perfectly natural for what you've just been through. But you'll feel far better than you did when you awoke to the beeps and buzzers of the intensive care unit, and you might even feel better than you did before your surgery, if you've had heart disease for some time. Heart disease advances slowly enough that often you don't notice the limits it has placed on your life until surgery removes them. You should see definite improvement each day for about the first six weeks following your surgery. After that, your progress is steady though less dramatic. Believe it or not, there'll come a time when you realize with a shock that oh, yes, you did have heart surgery once.

Red Alert! Pay attention to your body's messages as your recovery progresses. If it hurts, don't do it. Beware of sudden reaching (especially when you think you're ready to drive). If pain continues for longer than 30 minutes after you stop the activity that causes it, call your doctor. Also call your doctor if you experience sudden shortness of breath or chest pain, or if you notice redness and swelling around your incision.

When Does Life Get Back to Normal?

Everyone's idea of "normal" is unique. If yours is saddle-training horses, pass the reins to someone else for a spell. It takes about six months for your sternum (breastbone), which your surgeon has to cut to get to your heart, to heal completely. If you do something a little tamer for a living, you could well be back at it in two or three months. Most people, even horse trainers, can eventually return to the jobs and hobbies they enjoyed before surgery.

You'll return to routine life activities much sooner—driving in a few weeks, tee time on the golf course in a couple months. (Though if you plead your case with your doctor, you might get a note excusing you from housework for, oh, say, two, three years...) In time (six months to two years), that bold red scar on your chest will fade to a barely noticeable line.

Everything's Different!

What is this? The face staring back from the mirror looks like the same old face, but somehow everything's different. Bland foods taste salty, sour foods sweet, sweet foods intolerable. You're uncharacteristically emotional, crying over things you previously wouldn't even have noticed. You can't remember what happened the day you went to surgery or who came to visit you in the hospital the day or two after. Your family's confused and upset because you're not who you used to be. Try not to worry. These things are common aspects of recovery, and many are temporary (although some changes in taste linger).

It's not unusual for things to seem different after heart surgery. Your body *is* different, which you can sense more than see (except for that lovely work of art traversing your chest). It's had at least one near-death experience (when doctors stopped your heart to do surgery) or more (the heart attack that preceded surgery). You'll regain your emotional equilibrium as your body heals. Since heart disease develops gradually, quite possibly this is the first time in decades that your heart's been "well." As disorienting as these differences are at first, they're wonderful opportunities to adopt a heart-healthy lifestyle.

> **Cardio Care**
>
> Feeling down, even though you have every reason to be glad to be alive? Depression following a major trauma, such as a heart attack or heart surgery, is not uncommon. If you find yourself irritable, moody, disinterested in activities you once enjoyed, unable to sleep, and generally unhappy, let your doctor know. It often helps to talk with a counselor or to share your feelings with a support group.

When Is It Safe to Have Sex?

The first part of the answer is when your doctor says it is. Most doctors ask patients to let a week or two go by after leaving the hospital before they resume sexual activity. This is as much because your chest is still very tender as anything else. Many people worry that the strain of sexual activity will be more than their newly repaired hearts can stand. Not true. Can you climb a flight or two of stairs without stopping to rest, feeling winded, or having chest pain? Then your heart can handle sex. Sexual intercourse raises your pulse and blood pressure for a short time, but not high enough or long enough to cause damage—no more than climbing stairs.

Plan your return to sexual activity for a time when you're unrushed and well-rested, maybe in the morning when you're fresh instead of at night when you're tired from the day's activities. Let your body guide what you do and how fast you do it. Choose a position that avoids putting pressure on your sensitive incision (on your chest as well as on your leg if your doctor used a leg vein for your graft). If it hurts, don't do it. Your partner may be more worried than you are, fearing that in the throes of passion, something will happen. This is a common anxiety about an event that seldom happens. Yes, people do have heart attacks during sex. Just like they have them while walking the dog, carrying groceries in from the car, driving, and sleeping. Heart attacks actually brought on by sexual intercourse are rare.

Coping with Fears of Having Another Heart Attack

It's natural to worry about having another heart attack, especially if your first one seemingly came from nowhere. Having had a heart attack does increase your risk of having a second; the problems that set the stage don't go away, even with surgery. Consider your heart attack a wakeup call. Your heart has put you on notice that it's time for you to shape up… or it's shipping out.

Lifestyle changes are still the most significant part of your recovery. If you smoke, stop. Eat right, and exercise as your doctor instructs. Most heart surgery patients go through an outpatient cardiac rehabilitation program, which reinforces positive changes. A little fear is healthy; it keeps you aware of your actions and their possible consequences. But a life driven by fear is no fun for you or the people who share it with you. The best way to conquer fear is to focus on the positives. After all, you have a second chance at life! Focus on what you *can* do, not on what you can't.

Changing Your Life: One Day at a Time

While you were in the hospital, you received advice about nutrition, exercise, smoking, alcohol consumption, and other lifestyle issues. Now that you're on your own, how do you turn that advice into action? Most of us set goals that sound good but are nearly impossible to achieve because they're too big and negative. The habits that got your heart where it is evolved over many years, and developing new heart-healthy habits to replace them won't happen overnight. Set small, daily goals that you can reach. Make yourself a little chart, like the one that follows, each morning, and keep track of your progress. You'll be surprised at how much you accomplish, even when you feel like the only place you're going is nowhere fast.

Table 10.1 Sample Daily Plan

Today I Plan To	How I Did
Walk to the mailbox.	15 minutes each way
Eat a banana for breakfast.	Really wanted a donut, but the banana wasn't bad
Step outside, take a deep breath, and savor the fresh air.	Felt so good, did it three times
Take a short nap after lunch.	Laid down, couldn't fall asleep

After a while, many of these activities will just be part of your regular routine. Some will drop off (like naps), and others will grow (the walk to the mailbox might become a stroll to the corner, then around the block). Even if you haven't had heart surgery, this kind of daily plan can help you make heart-healthy changes in your lifestyle. And don't beat yourself up for slipping every now and then (though beware how quickly doing so slides into more often than not). Every day is a fresh start.

Beating the Odds

Heart surgery has become so successful, we expect its results to last forever. For some kinds of surgery, this is close to true. Valve replacements done today might well take you through the rest of your life. Other surgeries, like bypass grafts, have life expectancies of their own that may or may not coincide with yours. Before the mid-1990s, it was common to need another bypass operation 10 or 15 years after the first one. The new arteries eventually became clogged, too. New technology today is making repeat bypass surgery less likely. If your doctor detects a developing blockage early, balloon angioplasty might spare you another surgery. Also showing great promise is a device called a stent, a small, spring-like metal coil that the cardiologist can insert into an artery during angioplasty to help hold it open.

Just for YOU
Are you a smoker? Chances are you've been without a cigarette for a couple weeks by the time you come home from the hospital. Your addiction to nicotine worked its way out of your system while you were busy with other matters. Any cravings you have now are habit. Help yourself resist by having all evidence of smoking removed before you get home—cigarettes, ashtrays, lighters, and matches.

But technology can't fix the habits that cause heart disease in the first place. The American Heart Association warns that two out of three heart attack survivors fail to make the lifestyle changes that could extend their lives. One problem is that we don't see risks applying to us, even if we've already experienced them. In fact, having a heart attack and surviving may lead you to believe you're invincible—even if it happens again, you'll beat it because you did before. And you might. The longer we get away with "bad" habits, the less we believe in their badness. But your odds of living long enough to lecture your children and grandchildren about their lifestyles go way up if you eat right, exercise regularly, take your medications as directed, don't smoke, and pay attention to your heart's messages.

The Least You Need to Know

➤ Coronary bypass surgery is the most common and successful major surgery performed today.

➤ Most people who have heart surgery are back to their normal lives in two to three months.

➤ Physical addiction to nicotine ends between 48 hours and 10 days after your last cigarette. Since you've been without smoking all the time you've been in the hospital, the hard part's over. Stick with it, and enjoy the health benefits of smoke-free living.

➤ Changing habits takes time and effort. Reward yourself for the small successes. Take it one day at a time.

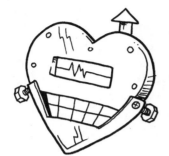

A New Heart for a New Century

The 21st century holds tantalizing promise for finding ways to end heart disease as we know it. We've come a long way since the introduction of the electrocardiograph in 1903 gave us a first peek at the intricate workings of the heart. Transplants, implants, and biogenetic technology make it possible to treat conditions in 1998 that once claimed hundreds of thousands of lives each year.

Looking for Magic

People born in the second half of the 20th century dodged many of the disease bullets that threatened people born in the first half. Between 1950 and today, medical science conquered, or at least thwarted, tetanus, polio, smallpox, cholera, the childhood disease quartet (measles, mumps, diphtheria, and chickenpox), influenza, and some forms of hepatitis. Antibiotics eliminate many bacterial infections. Now, we look to the wizard of medical magic, technology, to fix whatever ails us, even a "broken" heart.

Take It to Heart

South African surgeon Dr. Christiaan Barnard made medical history on December 3, 1967, when he removed the heart of a 23-year-old woman killed in a car accident and transplanted it into the chest of 55-year-old Louis Washkansky, whose heart disease left him barely able to handle the exertion of breathing. Washkansky lived 18 days before pneumonia claimed his life. Similar surgery on Dirk van Zyl, four years later, was extraordinarily successful. Van Zyl lived with his new heart for 23 years before dying of diabetes in 1994.

Heart Transplants

Each year, the ailing hearts of nearly 40,000 Americans reach the point where replacement becomes the sole hope for survival; 16,000 of those Americans are under the age of 55. Because donor hearts are hard to come by, only about 2,300 people get the new hearts they need. Immunosuppressive drugs developed in the early 1980s, combined with vastly improved surgical techniques, have made heart transplant surgery a successful treatment for those whose own hearts can no longer support them.

Just for YOU

Do you have a new heart? It's a marvel of the human body's ability to heal that within 6 months or so, the nerves of some people's transplanted heart begin to connect with their body's nervous system. Before long, the new heart can even feel pain (angina), restoring its "alert" system for letting you know it's not happy.

During an operation that takes about an hour, a heart-lung machine takes over the job of oxygenating your blood and sending it back out to your body while surgeons cut away your diseased heart. Surgeons leave the back portions of your atria (upper chambers). Surgeons trim the donor heart to fit onto this "stump," then sew the two pieces together. Most new hearts start beating by themselves as soon as warm blood enters them, though some need an electrical shock to "jump-start" them. A transplanted heart beats more quickly and responds more slowly to changes in demand, such as those created from exercise or exertion.

Heart transplants work best in people who are under the age of 60. If you have a heart transplant today, you have an 80 percent chance of making it through your first year after surgery and about a 40 percent chance of living 10 more years.

Organ rejection and infection remain the main threats following heart transplant surgery. After you have a heart (or other organ) transplant, you'll have to take immuno-suppressive drugs for the rest of your life to prevent your body from rejecting your new heart. Early immunosuppressive drugs were nonselective and simply turned off the entire immune system. This left transplant recipients extremely vulnerable to infection. Today's immunosuppressive drugs (like cyclosporin, azathio-prine, FK-506, and mycophenolate) prevent your immune system from attacking new organs, though they allow your immune system to go after other invaders. These drugs do have side effects, however, and you may end up taking additional medications to counter problems like hypertension, fluid retention, and tremors.

Surgeons performed about 38,000 heart transplants between 1967 and 1997. Like other sophisticated medical technology, heart transplants don't come cheap. A typical heart transplant costs close to $210,000 for surgery, the first year's drug treatment, and followup care. Each year after that runs about $15,000. Most major insurance companies cover these expenses—a sure sign that heart transplant is an accepted medical procedure, since insurers refuse to cover experimental treatment.

In Search of Donors

The main threat to a heart transplant is the severe shortage of donor hearts. Most organs for transplant come from people who die from trauma that results in severe brain injury, such as in car accidents, and have signed organ donor cards (on the back of your driver's license in many states), or their family members have given permission for organs to be removed for transplant.

The heart is the most fragile of all transplantable organs. For a successful transplant, doctors must remove a donor heart while it's still beating. Hospitals must often use breathing machines, or ventilators, to keep a donor's body alive after brain death occurs so surgeons have time to remove the heart. (Other organs, like livers, kidneys, and corneas, can be removed after the heart stops beating.) A new heart must be a near-perfect match with the recipient's tissue type (similar to blood type) to minimize the likelihood of rejection.

By Heart
Your immune system polices your body, always on the lookout for infections. It doesn't know your new heart is there to help, so it attacks the "intruder" in the same way it might attack a virus. This is called *organ rejection*, and without intervention, it will kill your new heart. Specialized *immunosuppressive drugs* fool your immune system into accepting your transplanted heart, preventing rejection.

Cardio Care
Want to give someone else the gift of life or sight when your life ends? Be an organ donor! Every year, 4,000 people die waiting for transplant organs. In many states, you can indicate your wish to be an organ donor on your driver's license. And tell your family that you want your organs donated, because they're the ones who'll have to sign the authorization forms.

High-Tech Biotech: Can You Clone a Heart?

If scientists can clone a sheep, can a human heart be far behind? On the 30-year anniversary of his historic surgery, heart transplant pioneer Dr. Barnard predicted that someday scientists will indeed "grow" human hearts. Genetic engineering techniques already in use allow laboratories to cultivate human skin from a few "starter" cells, a valuable aid for burn patients. But the heart is a far more complex organ. When developing naturally within a growing embryo, the heart starts as a simple tube-like pair of pumping pouches that go through several structural evolutions before becoming the four-chambered organ that sustains human life.

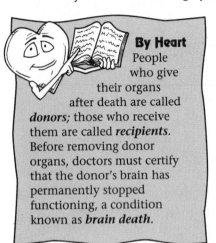

By Heart People who give their organs after death are called *donors;* those who receive them are called *recipients.* Before removing donor organs, doctors must certify that the donor's brain has permanently stopped functioning, a condition known as **brain death.**

For right now, cloning human organs is more a product of science fiction than science. But who knows what the next few decades hold? When you were born, would your parents have guessed that astronauts would shuttle to space and back, babies would start life in laboratories, and doctors would transplant human hearts?

Whatever Happened to the Artificial Heart?

A retired dentist, Barney Clark, earned his place in history in 1982 when he became the first person to receive a permanent artificial heart, a mechanical monstrosity called the Jarvik-7. Cumbersome and clumsy compared to the real thing, the Jarvik-7 replaced Clark's damaged heart with a mechanical pump powered by an external compressed-air system. Tubes through the chest wall connected the pump to the heart; the system's mechanical "beating" sounded more like wheezing. But the Jarvik-7 kept Clark alive for 112 days and gave renewed hope that scientists could find a way around the donor heart shortage.

Doctors soon realized that the artificial heart's limitations (size, power source, and infection risk) made it impractical as a permanent replacement for a damaged heart. A "normal" life would be next to impossible. Some researchers went back to the drawing board to try to design a mechanical heart and power supply small enough to fit entirely within the chest. Others turned their attention to adapting existing technology to meet other needs, such as temporary support for a failing heart. Over the next decade, both efforts achieved exciting results.

A modified design called a *left ventricular assistance device* (LVAD) emerged as a temporary "piggyback" support system to keep a damaged heart working long enough for doctors to find a replacement heart for transplant. The LVAD, smaller and more portable than its predecessors, attaches to the left ventricle and takes over pumping. Some people go as long as a year with an LVAD in place. LVADs are sometimes called *bridge* or *partial replacement pumps.* And new designs mean a completely internal mechanical heart will soon be available, powered by long-use batteries that will last five to ten years.

Take It to Heart

In 1994, Brazilian heart surgeon Dr. Randas Batista tried a radical approach to head off progressive heart damage in people with heart failure. In heart failure, your heart enlarges, unable to compensate for its inability to pump effectively. The larger your heart gets, the less effectively it pumps. Dr. Batista wondered what would happen if he simply made the heart smaller. So he tried cutting a wedge out of the enlarged left ventricle (pumping chamber), then sewing the edges together. Though it isn't the answer for everybody with heart disease, this still experimental procedure shows promise.

Closing In on the Causes of Heart Disease

Until recently, research has focused more on treating heart disease than preventing it. This is in part because most heart disease develops over many years, so testing ways to stop it would take a long time. People who already have heart disease don't have time to wait. Now, developments in treatment have opened new avenues of exploration for prevention.

We've known the factors that lead to heart disease for decades. But we haven't known just *how* heart disease happens—what actually causes blood pressure to go up or plaque to stick to the walls of your arteries. Recent studies of cell activity at the molecular level have revealed much information about how cells live, grow, reproduce, and die—and what can go wrong in the cycle. Researchers then translate this information into ways to prevent disease conditions from developing. Knowledge about how various proteins and enzymes affect cell metabolism, for example, often leads to new dietary recommendations.

Cardio Care

Medicare and many private insurers recently agreed to cover the cost ($70 to $80) of a new blood test that can check your homocysteine level. Homocysteine may be as important a factor in heart disease as cholesterol, and it is easier to control. Keep your homocysteine level low by increasing your vitamin B intake. Eat more fresh fruits and vegetables, or take a vitamin supplement.

Take Your Vitamins: Homocysteine and Heart Disease

"Eat your vegetables, they're good for you!" The timeless mantra of moms everywhere strikes a chord with today's researchers, who continue to discover new connections between health and vitamins. Always interested in getting to the bottom of what sounds like good advice, scientists started studying the relationship between vitamin levels and heart disease in the early 1970s. They found a surprising connection between B vitamins—B_6, B_{12}, and folic acid—and heart disease. People who had heart attacks also had low levels of folic acid. Further digging uncovered a likely culprit, the amino acid homocysteine.

Your body makes homocysteine when your cells metabolize proteins. As it turns out, homocysteine is a rather toxic waste product. In most people, other enzymes immediately swarm to neutralize it. In some people, however, these enzymes are a bit slow on the uptake—defective, in clinical terms. They allow homocysteine levels in the blood to remain very high. High homocysteine levels correlate with early, serious heart disease. A Harvard researcher actually discovered this correlation in 1974, but no one knew what to do about it, because no one knew what regulated homocysteine. Now, researchers know folic acid (a B vitamin) "feeds" the enzymes that attack homocysteine. A diet high in vitamin B keeps these enzymes hopping—and homocysteine levels low. Mom was right. Eat your fruits and vegetables (five servings a day). They're good for you… and your heart.

The following foods are a good source of most B vitamins (including folic acid). Cook vegetables lightly, if at all (microwave, steam, or stir-fry), to preserve their full load of vitamins.

Table 11.1 Foods High in B Vitamins

Asparagus	Lettuce
Beans (kidney, white, red, lima)	Mustard greens
Beets	Peas
Breakfast cereals (many have folic acid added)	Oranges and orange juice
Broccoli	Raspberries
Brussels sprouts	Soybean-based products (like tofu)
Bulgur (cracked wheat grains)	Spinach
Cauliflower	Wheat germ

Designer Genes

"I just can't help it" may become more truth than excuse as research into the role of genes in heart disease continues. While doctors have long known heart disease tends to run in families, they haven't been able to isolate the reasons. Do family members share unhealthy eating and exercise habits that make them more vulnerable to heart disease? Or is there more to the story? Recent research shows that genes may have far more control over conditions like heart disease than we previously thought.

Scientists already know genes cause a variety of other diseases, like muscular dystrophy, cystic fibrosis, and even *hypertrophic cardiomyopathy* (an overly muscular, severely enlarged heart). New studies have uncovered genes that may be responsible for a wide range of body responses, from fatty materials accumulating in your blood to sudden cardiac death. Doctors may someday be able to modify defective genes to prevent heart disease from developing or to change its course after it starts.

New Developments

One challenge in medical research is that no one knows how well new procedures and devices will work in human beings until they're used in real people. And most people aren't willing to gamble with their lives until it's the only chance they have for living. Sophisticated computer models give researchers a way to "see" their developments in simulated reality, helping them work out the bugs before using them in the real world. Other research is more speculative right now, examining the usefulness of technology such as cell transplants (now being tested for some forms of cancer) to treat damaged heart tissue.

Cardio Care
Rather than spending precious hours on the Web searching for the latest cures, take a walk in the park instead! Fresh air and exercise is a great combination for clearing your head and reducing stress (you can even take along some music to help you switch gears).

Coping in the 21st Century

Every week, it seems, there's a news report about a wonder drug or miracle treatment. How do you know what's true and what's important to you? This age of information is a mixed blessing. You can't afford to be uninformed. How much time do you spend shopping for a new television, computer, car, or even groceries? Do you double-check advertising claims, read technical reviews, compare labels? Your health deserves at least as much! Just because a procedure, test, or treatment is the latest thing, it's not necessarily the greatest. Or even good for you. Patients bombard doctors with requests for whatever is in the news, often without knowing the full story.

Here are three tips to help you sort through the confusion:

➤ **If it sounds too good to be true, it probably is.** This age-old saying is trite but valid. There are no quick fixes for most health problems. Prevention is seldom as simple as a pill or special drink. Unfortunately, we want to believe in magic, and we want to live forever. The combination makes us prime targets for modern "snake oil" remedies that may do more harm than good.

➤ **Not everything works for everybody.** Read the fine print (if you can find it). Legitimate medical tests and procedures include criteria (guidelines for use) that identify who or what conditions are likely to benefit. What difference will the information make? Knowing for the sake of knowing is interesting, but if what you learn makes no difference to how you'll live or what treatment approach you'll follow, it's relatively useless.

➤ **Consider the source.** The process of scientific study relies on verifiable, repeatable experiences. True medical breakthroughs receive wide attention and inspection. Researchers in Boston should be able to duplicate the results of researchers in San Francisco or Tokyo or London. Beware the common source, however. In today's high-tech environment, "news" reaches consumers almost instantly. One source quickly becomes dozens. Look for study descriptions to see if those seven articles all came from the same single report.

Red Alert!
Web-surfers, beware! Unlike medical journals that require proof of study findings, no one regulates the Web. Anyone can post anything. The Web contains vast amounts of misinformation. By all means, use the Internet to research health topics. Then verify the information you find through other independent sources, like journal articles (a librarian can guide you to sources). Talk with your doctor about material that seems relevant to you.

When you think a new test or treatment reported in the news could benefit you, schedule an appointment to talk it over with your doctor. Learn as much as you can, and take copies of articles with you. Don't stop what your doctor has recommended, or start something new on your own, until you have this discussion!

The information/technology explosion snares most doctors, too. They rely on a few trusted sources of information, like the American Heart Association, the American College of Physicians, and the *New England Journal of Medicine*. And, the *Wall Street Journal* and the *New York Times,* for example, are good sources for nonmedical, up-to-date information. If you come across a hot new tip, run it by your doctor, but don't be surprised if he or she needs to double-check the information. There are several thousand new medical articles published every week.

The Least You Need to Know

➤ A heart transplant is a successful, though limited, option for treating end-stage heart disease.

➤ A high level of homocysteine in your blood increases your risk for early heart disease. Lower your level—and your risk—by eating a diet high in folic acid.

➤ New technologies like gene therapy and cell transplants hold promise for thwarting the development of heart disease.

➤ You have more responsibility than ever before to be aware and informed about health matters that concern you. The more you learn about prevention, testing, and treatment for heart disease and other conditions, the better equipped you are to make the right decisions.

Part 3
The Way to Heart Health Is Through Your Stomach

Jack Sprat could eat no fat, His wife could eat no lean; And so betwixt them both, They licked the platter clean.

—Nursery rhyme

Ever feel like Jack and his wife live inside you? Americans spend nearly $700 billion on food each year, about 11 percent of the typical household income. Yes, we're eating more vegetables and fruits than ever before—each of us chows down nearly 700 pounds a year. But we're eating more added fat, too—65 pounds each in a year.

Sshhh! Hear that groaning? That's your heart. Most of us consume far more fat than is heart-healthy, and it shows—in the mirror and in the statistics. But you'll soon have your heart singing a happy tune, because the next four chapters tell you how to let the "Jack" in you control more of your diet.

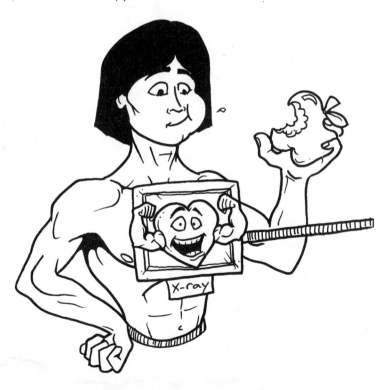

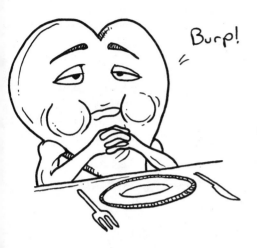

Burp!

A Full Heart

Since we no longer hunt or grow our own food (backyard gardens excepted), eating is as much a social event as a process of nourishing the body. Do you think about what effect that forkful of chocolate cake (or salad) will have once it enters your system? Most of us don't—our minds are on other things, like squeezing a few more minutes from a hectic morning or getting back to work on time after lunch. Yet the food choices we make—whether we think about them or not—shape more than just the body that looks back from the mirror.

Are Your Eyes Bigger Than Your Belly?

Appetite's a funny thing. You think it means you're hungry, but sometimes it's just telling you those fresh-baked cinnamon rolls smell good enough to eat. So you have one, whether or not you're actually hungry. Though we think of appetite and hunger as one

Just for YOU

Are you a woman under age 50 who weighs 30 percent more than you should? Your risk of heart disease is two and a half times that of a woman your age whose weight is within the desirable range. Your risk of high blood pressure is three times greater. Even a modest weight loss of 8 to 10 pounds lessens your risk. Combine heart-healthy eating habits with regular exercise to make your weight loss steady and permanent.

Cardio Care

Measure your waist at its narrowest point and your hips at their widest, then divide your waist measurement by your hip measurement. If the result is greater than .85 if you're a woman, or greater than 1 if you're a man, your fat-distribution pattern gives you higher health risks that you can lower by losing weight.

and the same, they're really quite different. Appetite feels good, combining the looks, smells, and memories of foods with the desire to partake of them. Hunger, on the other hand, is a rather unpleasant sensation your hypothalamus (a grape-sized region in your brain that controls autonomic or automatic nervous system activities) creates by telling your stomach to start churning. Generally, low blood sugar triggers this sequence of events, your body's signal that it needs nourishment. Appetite and pleasure, not hunger pains, tend to drive our eating habits.

"I Can't Believe I Ate the Whole Thing!"

Funny how all of a sudden that bag of chips or carton of ice cream just disappears. Vamoosed, gone, sucked right into thin air. Well, not quite thin air. (Is that chocolate on your chin?) More like down the hatch. What do you do when you eat? Besides move food from your plate to your mouth, that is. Do you read? Watch TV? Do you eat alone? Studies show that when you're doing something else while you eat, especially if you eat alone, you eat more.

Weighing In

Got one of those always-off-by-10-pounds scales in your bathroom? Must've been a special on them, as popular as they are! Truth is, 35 million Americans weigh at least 20 percent more than is healthy. If your ideal weight is 150 pounds and you weigh 185, for example, you're among them. Extra weight strains all your body systems, from your feet to your heart. Losing just 10 pounds can make a noticeable difference in your energy level and how you feel about yourself. And losing more, if that's what you need to do, has benefits far beyond appearance and feelings.

Table 12.1   Desired Weights of Women Aged Twenty-Five and Over

Height	Small Frame	Medium Frame	Large Frame
4'10"	102–111	109–121	118–131
4'11"	103–113	111–123	120–134
5'0"	104–115	113–126	122–137

Height	Small Frame	Medium Frame	Large Frame
5'1"	106–118	115–129	125–140
5'2"	108–121	118–132	128–143
5'3"	111–124	121–135	131–147
5'4"	114–127	124–138	134–151
5'5"	117–130	127–141	137–155
5'6"	120–133	130–144	140–159
5'7"	123–136	133–147	143–163
5'8"	126–139	136–150	146–167
5'9"	129–142	139–153	149–170
5'10"	132–145	142–156	152–173
5'11"	135–148	145–159	155–176
6'0"	138–151	148–162	158–179

Reprinted with permission of Metropolitan Life Insurance Company, Statistical Bulletin.

*Women between the ages of 18 and 25 should subtract one pound for each year under 25.

Table 12.2 Desired Weights of Men Aged Twenty-Five and Over

Height	Small Frame	Medium Frame	Large Frame
5'2"	128–134	131–141	138–150
5'3"	130–136	133–143	140–153
5'4"	132–138	135–145	142–156
5'5"	134–140	137–148	144–160
5'6"	136–142	139–151	146–164
5'7"	138–145	142–154	149–168
5'8"	140–148	145–157	152–172
5'9"	142–151	148–160	155–176
5'10"	144–154	151–163	158–180
5'11"	146–157	154–166	161–184
6'0"	149–160	157–170	164–188
6'1"	152–164	160–174	168–192
6'2"	155–168	164–178	172–197
6'3"	158–172	167–182	176–202
6'4"	162–176	171–187	181–207

Reprinted with permission of Metropolitan Life Insurance Company, Statistical Bulletin.

Height/weight charts give good general guidelines. But where you carry body fat could be more important than how much of it you're packing. If you're overweight and thick around the waist (an "apple" body shape), you're at higher risk for health problems, including diabetes, heart disease, and stroke. Extra weight that rides on your hips and thighs (a "pear" shape) doesn't seem to carry this added risk.

When Your Heart Can't Stand the Strain

Overindulgence at the table could easily turn a rich dinner into your last meal. A heart on the edge of obstruction (or that has already suffered damage in a heart attack) might limp along just fine until something challenges its blood supply—like that belt-loosening second or third (or fourth) helping. As your digestive system draws extra resources to help devour its heavy load, arteries, veins, and capillaries serving the organs participating in digestion (stomach, small intestine, pancreas, gallbladder, and liver) dilate to get more blood on the scene, bringing energy and taking nutrients away to feed other parts of the body.

Remember, your body is a closed system—you only have so much blood. What goes to your belly comes from other places, like your brain and your heart. Your brain handles the temporary shortage by sending signals to the rest of your body that it's nap time. A damaged heart (one with severely blocked arteries or scarring from previous heart attacks) has no retreat. When its blood supply drops, it quits.

So, What Do You Eat? (And How Much...): A Self-Quiz

Do you consult the food pyramid or the junk-food pile when making eating choices? Most of us have little idea of what we eat in a day, or how much of it. Take this short quiz to get a handle on your eating habits:

➤ I eat when...

    A. It's mealtime, whether I'm really hungry or not.

    B. I smell or see something good.

    C. I'm nervous or stressed, so pretty much all the time.

    D. When my body tells me it needs nourishment, whether it's a traditional mealtime or not.

➤ My idea of a serving size is...

    A. What the package or label says, if there is one.

    B. As much as my plate'll hold.

    C. More than what anybody else gets.

    D. Smaller than what I think I'll eat, because I know I can have more if I'm still hungry.

➤ I stop eating when...

    A. My plate's empty.

    B. I have to loosen my belt.

    C. I'd have to fix more to keep eating.

    D. I feel satisfied.

➤ My favorite pick-me-up snack is...

    A. Coffee, three sugars, double cream.

    B. Cookies and milk.

    C. Chips and dip followed by a candy bar.

    D. A glass of fresh, cold water and a piece of fruit.

➤ The food pyramid is...

    A. Something I can stand on to reach the shelf where the cookies are.

    B. An Egyptian memorial to a pharaoh who loved to eat.

    C. An elaborate scheme where the people at the bottom can't eat until the people at the top are full.

    D. Guidelines to help me make nutritious food choices.

If you selected D as your response to all the questions, you're probably on track with your daily diet. If you desperately wanted to choose Bs and Cs but didn't in case someone found your answers, pay particular attention to the next three chapters. And if you found yourself choosing A before moving on to read the rest of the answers, relax. You're only human!

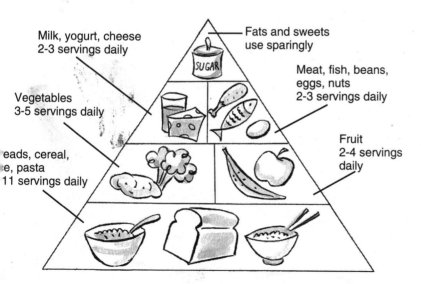

Milk, yogurt, cheese
2-3 servings daily

Fats and sweets
use sparetly

Meat, fish, beans,
eggs, nuts
2-3 servings daily

Vegetables
3-5 servings daily

Fruit
2-4 servings
daily

eads, cereal,
e, pasta
11 servings daily

The food pyramid illustrates the food groups that meet your body's nutritional needs. Choose plenty of foods from the bottom of the food pyramid; your body needs these the most. Choose fewer servings from food groups near the top of the pyramid; your body needs these the least.

Hey, What's Healthy, Anyway?

Seems like every time you turn on the news or pick up a paper, there's another report about something you've been eating all your life that's now bad for you. Just what *can* you eat? Well, it's hard to go wrong when you pick foods right from mother nature. Fruits and vegetables have no fat and plenty of vitamins. In general, the closer to nature your food is, the better it is for you.

Take It to Heart

If you've been out of school longer than you were in, you probably remember nutrition as "the four basic food groups." Look closely at the food pyramid, and you'll see that those familiar favorites are still there, just reorganized a bit. The federal *Food and Drug Administration* (FDA) developed the food pyramid in 1992 to reflect new information about nutrition and health.

Know Your Nutrients

Your body needs nourishment from six groups of essential nutrients:

➤ **Carbohydrates:** Sugars and starches provide energy for your body. About half of your daily diet should come from carbohydrates. Good sources of carbohydrates include cereals, grains, fruits, and products made from them (like bread and pasta).

➤ **Proteins:** These nutrients are made of amino acids, which your body needs for cell growth and repair. Good sources of protein include eggs, milk, cheese, poultry, and meat.

➤ **Fats:** The problem isn't that we eat fats—which our bodies need for energy—but that we eat too many foods high in fat. Fats should be no more than 20 to 30 percent of your daily diet (the average American diet is about 38 percent fat). Meats, dairy products, vegetable oils, fish, and avocados have high fat contents.

➤ **Fiber:** Even though your body can't digest fiber, it needs fiber to aid the digestive process by providing bulk. Good sources of fiber include raw fruits and vegetables, grains, and cereals.

➤ **Vitamins and Minerals:** These nutrients are essential for metabolism. Fruits, vegetables, grains, and cereals are especially good sources for vitamins and some minerals. Meats and poultry provide other minerals.

➤ **Water and Oxygen:** We don't always think of these substances as nutrients, but without them, your body couldn't survive. Every life function requires both water and oxygen. Your body is about 60 percent water. You should drink at least eight glasses of water daily.

Eating Too Much of the Wrong Things

Not everyone who weighs more than they should eats too much. Other factors sometimes play a role, like genetics and, less commonly, disease conditions.

Take It to Heart

Are you an ectomorph, endomorph, or mesomorph? These three body types may have more to do with how much you weigh than your diet or activity level. Ectomorphs, for example, have lean, small frames and low fat-storage capacity. Endomorphs have rounded, larger frames and can store equally large amounts of fat. Muscular mesomorphs are in-between. If you're an endomorph, you're not likely to ever look as slight as an ectomorph—even one who's the same weight and height.

How Much Should You Eat?

It's not easy to know how much is enough. The average person (someone not trying to lose weight) needs 1,500 to 2,000 calories a day. We all know those extra calories lead to body fat, but at what point do we cross the line? Here's a handy formula to help you figure out how many calories your daily diet should contain:

1. Weigh yourself (no clothes, no cheating).
2. Multiply your weight by 15. This gives you the number of calories (average) that you use each day to stay at your current weight.
3. To lose weight at the rate of one to two pounds a week (recommended), multiply your weight by 12. This gives you the number of calories you should eat each day, on average, for a slow and steady weight loss.
4. Maintain your new weight by taking in 15 times your weight in calories each day.

Take It to Heart

One pound equals 3,500 calories. The most effective way to lose weight and keep it off is to reduce your daily calorie intake by 500 calories. This leaves you enough food to feel satisfied, yet knocks off a pound a week (500 calories × 7 days = 3,500 calories = 1 pound). Combine calorie reductions with increased exercise for improved fitness and faster results.

Developing Healthy Eating Patterns

One of the best things about "good" foods is that they tend to squelch your appetite for junk foods over time. Foods with substance to them—fruits, vegetables, grains—encourage (and sometimes require!) you to chew them slowly and completely. This releases chemicals in your mouth and stomach, setting in motion the chain of events that eventually will tell your brain you're full. You can't chew junk food this thoroughly—there's not enough there. Go ahead, put a French fry or doughnut through 15 or 20 chews. You won't have much left but mush by the fourth or fifth chomp, and that won't satisfy your mouth or your brain.

Cardio Care

If you eat a vegetarian diet, be sure you get plenty of vitamin C, which helps your body absorb iron and other minerals from plant sources. Also include a wide variety of grains, beans, nuts, and seeds to be sure you get enough protein. Rice and beans (red, lima, pinto, and similar types) together, for example, form a good source of protein.

Heart-Healthy Diets

Stop thinking of "diet" as something you do and start thinking of it as a way of life! It's hard to make changes when you think of what you're doing as depriving yourself of pleasures you really enjoy. The more healthful foods you eat, the more they'll replace those unhealthy pleasures. Eventually, that cheeseburger you just can't live without becomes intolerably heavy and greasy, a jolt of taste sensations your mouth no longer finds appealing. Remember, most tastes are acquired. You're not born loving those cheeseburgers. You can change your tastes (it takes about three or four weeks to "reprogram" your taste buds), and you might be surprised how much better you like the new ones.

To Help Prevent Heart Trouble

The earlier you start heart-healthy eating habits, the bigger the payoff in terms of preventing heart problems. But it's never too late to change. These suggestions might help you smooth your transition to a heart-healthy diet:

➤ Plan your meals, including snacks. Buy only the food items you need to prepare them.

➤ Choose foods you like from among the six categories, with the food pyramid as your guide. Include all categories among each day's food choices.

➤ Try different foods and different seasonings. "Variety's the very spice of life," said William Cowpers. Variety is also the heart of a healthy diet.

➤ Find practical substitutes for high-fat favorites. Do you like sour cream on your baked potato? Try low-fat plain yogurt instead. Have a few low-salt pretzels instead of a handful of chips. Be creative—your options are endless!

➤ Find foods you like. Can't stand lima beans, and broccoli makes you gag? Don't eat them. Eat other vegetables that provide the same nutrients. Supermarkets carry an incredible variety of produce.

To Help Reverse Heart Trouble

Reversing heart trouble through diet (in combination with regular exercise) requires a strong commitment to change. Most diets to reverse heart disease are vegetarian, to reduce dietary fat to an absolute minimum. Such diets are typically low in salt as well. If you decide to try this approach, talk with your doctor or a nutritionist about how to get the nutrients your body needs from a vegetarian diet.

And don't forget the rest of you. Your heart disease–reversal program needs elements for each aspect of your whole being—diet and exercise for your physical body, meditation or prayer for your spiritual being, and stress-reduction methods to achieve emotional balance.

By Heart
A vegetarian diet excludes meat. A meatless diet that includes dairy products and some poultry and fish is called *semivegetarian.* A meatless diet that includes milk and eggs, but no fish or poultry, is called *lacto-ovovegetarian;* one that excludes eggs as well is called *lactovegetarian.* A *vegan* diet is the strictest form of vegetarian diet and excludes all animal products, including eggs and dairy.

"But I Don't Want to Change the Way I Eat!"

You don't *have* to change the way you eat, of course. After all, you've lived just fine this long. You may well live lots longer. (And you could rip the plaster off your walls to remodel and find bundles of money tucked between the studs. Hey, it happens!) If your eating habits are leading you to an early heart attack but you don't want to change them, it's time for a little chat with yourself. What is it, exactly, that you don't want to change? Why? Do you like the way those greasy cheeseburgers taste, slide down your throat with minimal help from your teeth, save a few bucks on lunch expenses? Or do you just like the guys at the burger place?

While there's not a whole lot you can do to make a cheeseburger heart-healthy, many restaurants (even burger places) offer menu selections not quite so high in fat. The truth is, a double burger with cheese and the works can by itself exceed the American Heart Association's recommended guidelines for fat (30 percent or less of your daily calories). Consider these options to make changing your eating habits more palatable:

➤ Walk to and from your favorite burger spot, walk around the block before you go in, or at least park at the end of the lot and walk briskly to the door.

➤ Eat your favorite burger on, say, Tuesdays and Thursdays, and eat salads or stir-fry the rest of the week. You'll still have high fat intake two days a week, but over the course of the week, you could average out to the recommended level.

➤ Hold the mayo, add mustard, toss on some lettuce and tomatoes, try a whole wheat bun. Not that we want to destroy the great taste you've grown to love, but every little bit helps.

If you really can't bring yourself to make any changes in the way you eat, start collecting the names of cardiologists your friends and neighbors recommend. You're going to need one sooner than you think.

The Least You Need to Know

➤ Appetite, not hunger, drives our eating habits. While hunger is a physiological (bodily) response, appetite is learned.

➤ Diet is a way of life, not just a way to lose weight.

➤ What crosses your lips shapes the health of your heart, not just the size of your hips.

➤ For optimal results, combine a heart-healthy diet with regular exercise. Your heart'll thank you!

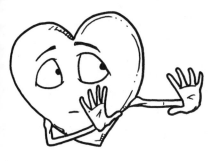 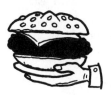

Chapter 13

No Fat, Low Fat, Whoa... Fat!

In This Chapter

➤ Why we need fat

➤ The different kinds of fat

➤ Reading and comparing food labels

➤ Making low-fat food choices

Odd as it sounds, we eat fat because we like how it tastes. Not by itself, usually, but in other foods. Fat gives fried chicken, French fries, and potato chips their crispy crunch. It also gives chocolate its smoothness and cakes their fluffy texture. Fat is everywhere in our eating habits. Is this bad? It depends. Your body needs a certain level of dietary fat to function. But most of us consume far more fat than our bodies need. A high-fat diet causes problems, for your wardrobe and for your heart.

Take It to Heart

The scientific community uses metric units of measurement, so food-label information appears in grams and milligrams. This can get confusing when portion sizes are in ounces. A quick conversion is about 28 grams to an ounce. An ounce of fat contains about 252 calories, while an ounce of protein or carbohydrate has about 112. A tablespoon is roughly equal to half an ounce, so a tablespoon of something that's all fat, like butter or margarine, contains about 126 fat calories.

Why Do We Need Fat, Anyway?

With all the negative press fat gets, you'd think the stuff was just bad for you, period. Not so. Fatty foods supply fat-soluble vitamins—like A, D, E, and K—that your body needs for cell metabolism and tissue repair. Dietary fat also provides energy. A single gram of fat provides nine calories, compared to four or five calories in a gram of carbohydrates. In cultures in which people hunt and gather their food from day to day, body fat is a ready store of energy for those times when food is scarce. In contemporary Western culture, however, most of the hunting and gathering we do takes place at the supermarket.

How Much Fat Is Enough Fat?

Dietary fat becomes a problem when it accounts for more than its share of calories. Your body starts looking for places to store its extra reserve. Some you notice right away, like your waist and hips. Your body has about 40 billion fat cells it can call into action. Once this energy buffer doubled as insulation to protect your body from external temperature extremes. Today, we have extensive wardrobes to take over this role. Extra fat stored in this way is, well, just added weight. Other deposits are less obvious (and more harmful), like in your arteries. As these deposits accumulate, they begin to restrict the flow of blood. This can lead to a stroke or heart attack.

The American Heart Association recommends a diet that gets fewer than 30 percent of its calories from fat. The typical American diet contains about 38 percent fat. Three in ten Americans tip the scales at 20 percent above their ideal (and healthy) weight.

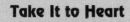

Take It to Heart

Contrary to popular belief, gaining weight doesn't cause your body to add fat cells. Your body's fat cells function rather like balloons. When empty, fat cells are collapsed, like balloons in the package. When your body sends excess fat to them, they fill—like removing balloons from the package and blowing them up. When you lose weight, the emptied cells collapse again—like letting the air out of a balloon and putting it back in the package. They're still there, though, ready (whenever you are) to fill up again.

East Meets West

More than half of the world's population eats a diet that is primarily vegetarian. Because they exclude meat, vegetarian diets are naturally low in fat (though certain fruits, like olives and avocados, and most nuts and seeds have a very high fat content). Look again at the food pyramid in Chapter 12, "A Full Heart."

A diet rich in grains, vegetables, and fruits (along with milk products to provide calcium and vitamin D) easily fulfills daily standards for essential nutrients. In many Asian countries, for example, a traditional diet contains mostly rice, vegetables, chicken, and fish. Few dishes are fried. Such a diet includes only about 9 or 10 percent fat—and coronary artery disease is far less common.

Sometimes "translating" these foods to American plates makes them more high-fat disaster than low-fat delicacy. Yes, Chinese, Japanese, Thai, Korean, Vietnamese, and other Eastern-culture dishes can be heart-healthy additions to your diet—as long as you don't bread them, fry them, or smother them in sugary sauces. It's quite possible to go out for what you think is a low-fat meal and end up consuming three days' worth of fat and cholesterol through careless menu choices.

Why a Low-Fat Diet Is Heart Healthy

It's sometimes hard to understand why fat's such a big deal. If it tastes so good, how can it be so bad for your body? Two reasons, actually, and neither has anything to do with taste (which, remember, is a learned behavior). You just finished Chapter 12, so you know your body uses different essential nutrients in different ways. In some ways, it's like pegs and holes—your body never uses vitamins to fill a carbohydrate's function. A diet too high in fat cheats your heart in two ways. First, it keeps those 40 billion or so fat cells pretty busy. This gives your heart more body surface to supply with blood.

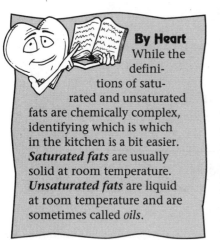

By Heart
While the definitions of saturated and unsaturated fats are chemically complex, identifying which is which in the kitchen is a bit easier. *Saturated fats* are usually solid at room temperature. *Unsaturated fats* are liquid at room temperature and are sometimes called *oils*.

Second, a diet high in fat is likely low in other essential nutrients, especially those that come from low-fat sources like grains, vegetables, and fruits. Sure, your body still works just fine—now (as far as you can tell). And you could run heavy-weight motor oil in your new car, too. After all, 20W50 worked just fine in those old V-8s you drove until you got this little four-banger, which seems to be doing OK with it, too (what does the idiot who wrote the owner's manual know, anyway?). But eventually your car's engine, like your heart on a high-fat diet, is going to start complaining. You'll go out to crank it over one morning, and pffttt! That's all she wrote. Need a new engine, you're out maybe $1,000 and a week while your car's in the shop. Need a new heart, you're out of—time? Luck? Life?

Here a Fat, There a Fat...

Finding fat isn't as simple as you'd think. For one thing, there's more than one kind of fat. Each comes from a different source and has a different effect in (and on) your body. Some fats are obvious, like butter and the white stuff surrounding that New York cut you're about to slap on the grill. Others lurk within foods like meat, fish, and poultry.

Most fats fall into one of two categories: *saturated* and *unsaturated*. Ready for a brief return trip to chemistry 101? Fats, at the chemical level, contain carbon, hydrogen, and a touch of oxygen. What separates saturated fats from unsaturated fats is the hydrogen. Saturated fats are full, chemically speaking, with each carbon atom paired to a hydrogen atom. When two or more carbon atoms lack hydrogen partners, the fat is unsaturated. *Polyunsaturated fats* are unsaturated fats with many solo carbon atoms.

All this becomes important during metabolism, because hydrogen atoms prevent your body from breaking down fats into other substances. Think about it like pairing up for dancing. Saturated fats come to the dance already holding hands, unwilling to part with each other.

Saturated Fat

If saturated fats have a motto, it's "from the lips to the hips." These fats come from animals and make their way into your diet as meat (like steak, pork, bacon, lamb, sausage, and lunchmeat), milk, cheese, butter, and lard. They come aboard flashing express tickets right to your fat cells, since their chemical structure prevents your body from breaking them down into other substances.

If saturated fats just went to your fat cells and stayed there, they might not do much damage except to your image. Unfortunately, they leave fragments of fatty material along the walls of your arteries, like microscopic skid marks. Over time, these build into blockages. (Maybe that motto should be "from the lips to the arteries.")

Saturated fats also contribute to your body's level of *low density lipoprotein* (LDL) cholesterol. There is a direct relationship between LDL levels and coronary artery disease. (We talk about cholesterol in Chapter 14, "How Does Cholesterol Count?") No more than 10 percent of your total daily calories should come from saturated fats.

Unsaturated Fat

Unsaturated fats come primarily from plants—corn, olives, soybeans, and sunflowers are common sources. They show up in your diet as oils (often in a homogenous form simply called *vegetable oil*). Unsaturated fats are better for your heart, because they don't raise your LDL (though they do still accumulate in your fat cells). No more than 20 percent of your total daily calories should come from unsaturated fats.

Trans–Fatty Acids

Some unsaturated fats use a process called *hydrogenation* to add consistency to a product that would otherwise be fairly liquid. Solid cooking oils and stick margarines are good examples of partially hydrogenated fats. Hydrogenation also produces trans–fatty acids (sometimes called trans-fats).

Scientists suspect that trans–fatty acids play a role in raising LDL cholesterol, possibly contributing to clogged arteries. The harder the product, the higher the amount of trans–fatty acids. Stick margarines can contain 10 to 12 percent trans–fatty acids. Research continues about the health effects of trans–fatty acids. The best guideline is moderation. The foods most likely to contain trans-fats are also foods that don't contribute much to your diet beyond taste and calories. Many baked goods, especially those purchased ready-to-eat, are high in trans-fats because of the shortening they contain. French fries (cooked in vegetable oil) and snack foods also contain trans–fatty acids.

Cardio Care
Concern about the role trans–fatty acids play in clogged arteries and heart disease raised questions about the wisdom of substituting margarine, which contains trans–fatty acids in the form of partially hydrogenated fat, for butter, which contains saturated fat. The American Heart Association holds that saturated fat is the greater risk for heart disease and recommends selecting margarines that list vegetable oil as the first ingredient.

Just for YOU
Are you among the 38 million Americans who need to lose weight? If you reduce the amount of fat in your diet, the odds are high that you'll also reduce your overall calorie intake. When you count fat instead of just calories, you're taking the first important step toward making diet a way of life instead of short-term torture.

Fat-Free Doesn't Mean You Won't Gain Weight!

Sounds like a dream come true, doesn't it? No fat, eat all you want. Wake up! It's just a dream, and it's not true. While fat has more calories per gram than carbohydrates and proteins, these other nutrients still have calories. Fat calories take the lips-to-hips express route to fat cells. Other nutrients take the metro route, stopping at various metabolic stations along the way as your body first tries to use them for direct energy. When there are no takers, your body turns those extra calories to fat—by this stage, it doesn't matter in what food form they started. This fat shows up on your scale and in your mirror.

Reading and Comparing Food Labels

Federal regulations require food labels to contain certain information showing the product's complete ingredients and selected nutritional values.

Here's a food label from a cereal box.

Nutrition Facts

Serving Size 1 cup (30g)
Servings Per Container About 14

Amount Per Serving	Cheerios	with ½ cup skim milk
Calories	110	150
Calories from Fat	15	20
	% Daily Value**	
Total Fat 2g*	3%	3%
Saturated Fat 0g	0%	3%
Polyunsaturated Fat 0.5g		
Monounsaturated Fat 0.5g		
Cholesterol 0mg	0%	1%
Sodium 280mg	12%	15%
Potassium 95mg	3%	9%
Total Carbohydrate 22g	7%	9%
Dietary Fiber 3g	11%	11%
Soluble Fiber 1g		
Sugars 1g		
Other Carbohydrate 18g		
Protein 3g		
Vitamin A	10%	15%
Vitamin C	10%	10%
Calcium	4%	20%
Iron	45%	45%
Vitamin D	10%	25%
Thiamin	25%	30%
Riboflavin	25%	35%
Niacin	25%	25%
Vitamin B₆	25%	25%
Folic Acid	25%	25%
Vitamin B₁₂	25%	35%
Phosphorus	10%	25%
Magnesium	8%	10%
Zinc	25%	30%
Copper	2%	2%

*Amount in Cereal. A serving of cereal plus skim milk provides 2g fat (0.5g saturated fat, 1g monounsaturated fat), less than 5mg cholesterol, 350mg sodium, 300mg potassium, 28g carbohydrate (7g sugars) and 7g protein.

**Percent Daily Values are based on a 2,000 calorie diet. Your daily values may be higher or lower depending on your calorie needs:

	Calories:	2,000	2,500
Total Fat	Less than	65g	80g
Sat Fat	Less than	20g	25g
Cholesterol	Less than	300mg	300mg
Sodium	Less than	2,400mg	2,400mg
Potassium		3,500mg	3,500mg
Total Carbohydrate		300g	375g
Dietary Fiber		25g	30g

➤ **Serving size:** What the manufacturer considers to be a typical portion.

➤ **Servings per container:** How many portions the package holds. Further nutritional information is for each serving.

➤ **Calories/calories from fat:** Total calories in each serving, and how many calories in each serving come from fat.

➤ **Total fat:** Amount of fat, measured in grams, each serving contains. Also identifies what portion is saturated fat and what percentage of daily value (may appear on food labels as % Daily Value or %DV) this constitutes.

➤ **Cholesterol:** Amount of cholesterol, measured in milligrams, that each serving contains and what percentage of daily value this constitutes.

➤ **Sodium:** Amount of sodium, measured in milligrams, that each serving contains and the percentage of daily value this constitutes.

➤ **Total carbohydrate:** Amount of carbohydrates, measured in grams, that each serving contains and the percentage of daily value this constitutes. Under this, the label lists the relative amounts of dietary fiber and sugars in the carbohydrate.

➤ **Protein:** Amount of protein, measured in grams, that each serving contains.

➤ **Vitamin A, Vitamin C, Calcium, Iron:** Percentages of these substances each serving contains.

Food labels also include a chart demonstrating relative values of the substances the label reports for a typical diet of 2,000 (women) and 2,500 (men) calories. Remember that all reported information is per serving. Some packaging is misleading; how often do you eat half a candy bar or drink half a bottle of a sports drink? If the packaged meal you're about to have for lunch has 12 grams of fat, that's good—about 18 percent of your daily allotment. If half of that fat's saturated, though, that's not so good—there goes a third of your daily limit for saturated fat. Reading and comparing food labels helps you make informed (and heart-healthy) choices.

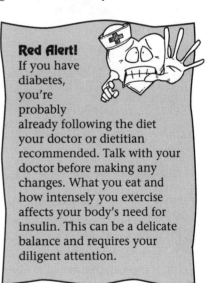

Red Alert!
If you have diabetes, you're probably already following the diet your doctor or dietitian recommended. Talk with your doctor before making any changes. What you eat and how intensely you exercise affects your body's need for insulin. This can be a delicate balance and requires your diligent attention.

Calculating Your Percentage of Calories from Fat

In Chapter 12, you calculated the total calories your diet should contain for your weight (actual or ideal, if you want to lose weight). To be absolutely precise in figuring out what percentage of those calories can come from fat, multiply your total by .30 (reflecting the American Heart Association's dietary recommendation of 30 percent). Those of you who are mathematically challenged can come close enough by dividing your daily calorie total by 3. Say, for example, that your weight is 160 pounds. You should take in about 2,400 calories a day to maintain that weight ($160 \times 15 = 2,400$). Thirty percent of your 2,400 calories is 720 calories—the precise amount of calories in your diet that should come from fat. Or, you can estimate your fat percentage by dividing by 3—800 calories.

As you can see, your estimate is somewhat higher than your precise percentage. For most people, the difference is not that significant—just 80 calories a day in our example. But beware! Those extra calories add up, whether or not you can do the math. In a month and a half, they become a full pound of fat—eight pounds in a year. (Talk about your heavy heart!) For those 80 fat calories, you could have three-fourths of a chocolate bar, two Oreo cookies, or seven potato chips. Or you could go the no-fat route for those same 80 calories and choose an apple, banana, or orange.

Cardio Care

Red meat is such a part of American life that many athletes believe they have to eat plenty of it to get the protein they need for strength and endurance. While an occasional red-meat meal is fine, chicken, turkey, tuna and other fish, pasta, and rice are all heart-healthy sources of protein. (Beans, too, though you might find their digestive side effects less than socially acceptable.)

Watch Out for Sugar!

Some products designed to be fat-free substitutes for their fat-bearing counterparts, like pastries and cookies, instead contain higher amounts of carbohydrates and sugars to make them taste better. One reason fats are so popular in Western culture is that they add flavor and texture to foods. Fat and heat, for example, combine to turn ordinary potatoes into that all-American delight, the potato chip. Removing fat from the formula often removes the taste, too—at least the taste we've grown to know and love. So many low-fat snack foods add the next-best thing: sugar.

What About Fat Substitutes?

Can it really be? A no-fat "fat?" In 1996, the FDA approved a no-calorie substitute for the fat used in snack foods called *olestra*. Products made with olestra fool your mouth, because olestra provides the same texture and taste as traditional fat. Though olestra is new on the market, food manufacturers have explored fat substitutes since the 1960s. Until olestra, such products featured a carbohydrate or protein base. They can't quite mimic the feel and flavor real fat adds to foods, however, and can't be used for frying.

Olestra is a fat-based product, so it behaves exactly like fat—with one important difference. Olestra's molecules are too big for your body to digest in the time it takes for an olestra-containing product to pass through your digestive system. So that's exactly what olestra does—pass through (though your body does digest the other substances in the product, like carbohydrates). At present, the FDA limits olestra to use in what it calls "savory snacks" like potato chips. Olestra appears to interfere with your body's ability to absorb fat-soluble vitamins (A, D, E, and K), so the FDA requires manufacturers of products containing olestra to add those vitamins.

Making Low-Fat Choices: A Self-Quiz

Do you know which food choices are low in dietary fat? Test yourself with this quick quiz! For each item, select the food that's lower in fat:

1. A cheeseburger or a tuna-salad sandwich?
2. Broiled salmon or broiled chicken breast?
3. Carob or milk chocolate?
4. Two eggs or two slices of bacon?
5. French fries or a baked potato?
6. A bottle of beer or a glass of wine?
7. A bagel with cream cheese or a roast-beef sandwich?
8. Granola or a doughnut?
9. Chocolate fudge or milk chocolate?
10. Lobster or filet mignon?

How'd you do? Check your answers!

1. The obvious choice seems to be the tuna, but don't pat yourself on the back yet. While tuna itself gets only 6 calories per serving from fat, the mayonnaise most tuna salad contains gets all its calories (100 per tablespoon) from fat. A cheeseburger made with extra-lean beef and low-fat cheese, served on a whole-wheat bun, could be a reasonable choice. But don't make this a daily menu item, and hold the mayo!

2. Salmon gets about a fourth of its calories from fat, just about the same as a chicken breast with skin. Strip the skin, though, and you drop almost half the fat calories. White-fleshed fish like cod, perch, orange roughy, and haddock get fewer than 10 percent of their calories from fat.

3. Carob and milk chocolate have about the same number of total and fat calories. Indulge your taste for either sparingly, and choose carob only if you really like it better than chocolate.

4. Eggs get 80 percent of their calories from fat, about a third of it saturated. Bacon gets 23 percent of its calories from fat, about 40 percent of it saturated. Neither of these foods is inherently bad; it's just that we tend to eat them often and in combination with each other.

5. French fries weigh in at 20 to 40 percent fat, depending on who makes them; about a third of that is saturated fat. A plain baked potato has no fat. All that stuff you put on it—butter, sour cream, bacon bits, maybe cheese sauce—can jack the fat content of your side dish way over that of those fries. Use low-fat alternatives to top your baker, and your heart'll sing your praises.

6. Ounce for ounce, alcohol has the same calories. Though none of them come from fat, your body quickly turns them into fat because they have no other nutritional value. Moderation, moderation!

7. Cream cheese more than makes up for the minimal fat calories in a bagel, with 90 percent of its calories from fat (60 percent of them saturated). A lean roast-beef sandwich, on the other hand, gets just 10 percent of its calories from fat. Just hold the mayo on that sandwich!

8. Granola comes in at about 20 percent fat, though some brands are much higher. A plain cake doughnut gets 25 percent of its calories from fat. Again, it's what you usually eat with it that makes the difference. Do you have that granola with whole or skim milk? Do you dress up that doughnut with chocolate frosting or cream filling?

9. Chocolate fudge may have the reputation for sinful deliciousness, but plain old chocolate takes the cake on this one. Chocolate gets about 35 percent of its calories from fat, and 85 percent of those are saturated. Fudge looks lean by comparison, with 18 percent of its calories from fat, though 37 percent of them are saturated.

10. Filet mignon comes from the grill to your table with 75 percent of its calories from fat, compared to a mere 16 percent for lobster. Unfortunately, not many people eat their lobster plain. That favorite dipping delicacy, drawn butter, is all fat, about 70 percent of it saturated. Is your favorite splurge these two together? (That scream you hear is your heart!)

Sometimes what appears to be the healthier choice isn't. While what foods you eat is important, how you prepare them sometimes matters more. High-fat toppings like butter, cheese, and bacon pieces can turn what starts as a heart-healthy meal into a cardiac nightmare.

Low- and No-Fat Foods Even You Can Love

Who wants to go through life eating food with all the flavor of cardboard? No one we know! Many people complain that a low- or no-fat diet is bland and boring. What do they know? You know better, because you're reading this book and we're going to tell you how to make your low-fat lifestyle zing!

Table 13.1 Fat Substitutions

Instead of...	Try...
Fried	Broiled, baked, poached, or steamed; use a fat-free spray to coat pans instead of margarine or cooking oil

Instead of...	Try...
Steak	Chicken or fish, or extra-lean broiled steak
French fries	Baked potato (see next item) or sliced potatoes baked with seasonings and a small amount of olive oil
Butter, sour cream, and bacon bits	Seasoned pepper and low-fat yogurt
Mayonnaise on sandwiches	Mustard, ketchup, low-fat honey-mustard dressing, pickles, tomatoes, lettuce, peperoncinis, green or red peppers, hot peppers, horseradish
Mayonnaise in salads	Low-fat mayonnaise, sandwich spread, vinegar, Worcestershire sauce, lemon or lime juice
Doughnuts	Muffins and bagels
Jams and jellies	Fruit spreads (low in sugar)
Salad dressings	Basalmic or flavored vinegars
Beef or pork sausage	Turkey or chicken sausage

Heart-healthy alternatives are no longer the exception in most grocery stores, restaurants, and even bakeries. Remember, eating is mostly habit. Once you make the switch to low-fat, you might be surprised how much you like the variety of your choices.

The Least You Need to Know

➤ Entirely no fat is no good. Your body needs fat-soluble vitamins and some dietary fat to function, and it stores fat to meet future energy needs.

➤ A low-fat diet reduces the buildup of fatty deposits in your arteries (plaque), lowering your risk of heart disease.

➤ Food labels provide a wealth of information to help you make heart-healthy choices.

➤ Low-fat doesn't have to be bland or boring. Experiment with different spices and combinations to replace high-fat favorites. Give your taste buds time to adjust.

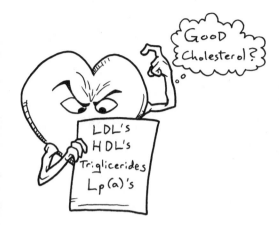

How Does Cholesterol Count?

What's all this fuss over cholesterol, anyway? Our great-grandparents didn't worry about what happened to food after they ate it, so why should we? Well, for starters, they didn't know about cholesterol or many other risk factors for heart disease. Now that we know about them, we can make heart-healthy decisions. And because of all this new medical knowledge, you're likely to live longer than your great-grandparents were when they died. Advances in medical technology have made long life not only possible but also enjoyable—if you take responsibility for your part. Now, you can bury your head in the past and pretend cholesterol doesn't matter. Or you can take control of one more risk factor to reduce the chance that heart disease will end your life.

Does a High Cholesterol Count Matter to Your Heart?

Doctors have known for many years that there's a strong connection between high blood cholesterol levels, atherosclerosis, and heart attacks. Just how this connection works remains a mystery, though. Some people with low blood cholesterol levels have heart attacks. And some people whose blood cholesterol levels are sky-high enjoy long and

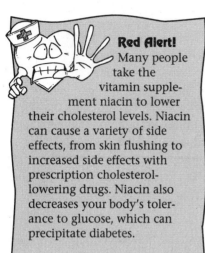

Red Alert! Many people take the vitamin supplement niacin to lower their cholesterol levels. Niacin can cause a variety of side effects, from skin flushing to increased side effects with prescription cholesterol-lowering drugs. Niacin also decreases your body's tolerance to glucose, which can precipitate diabetes.

By Heart What you've eaten recently can influence the levels of some substances, like triglycerides. Your doctor orders your blood to be drawn after you *fast*—you have no food for 12 to 14 hours before the test. Labs generally draw fasting tests first thing in the morning, so you can return to a normal eating schedule as your day begins. Total and HDL cholesterol levels do not require fasting.

apparently disease-free lives. Both extremes are exceptions, however. For most people, the more fatty material that accumulates in your arteries, the higher your chance of having a heart attack or stroke. Dietary cholesterol feeds that accumulation.

How Is Cholesterol Measured, and What's Normal?

A blood test shows your cholesterol level. Doctors typically order readings for total cholesterol and HDL (high density lipoprotein) or "good" cholesterol for screening purposes. If your total level is high and your HDL level is low, your doctor may order additional tests to get a better idea of what's going on. This is usually a fasting cholesterol panel, which includes total, HDL and LDL (low density lipoprotein) or "bad" cholesterol, and triglycerides. If your results are borderline, your doctor might have you try some lifestyle changes for a couple months, then repeat the blood test. Diet, exercise, and weight loss can drop cholesterol levels. The lab reports your cholesterol measurements as milligrams (mg) per deciliter (dl).

Table 14.1 Total Cholesterol Levels

Desirable	Less than 200mg/dl
Borderline high	200–239mg/dl
High	240mg/dl or higher

Your total cholesterol level is only a starting point, however. You need to know your HDL and your LDL to know where you really stand. The higher your HDL, the better. In fact, if your HDL is over 60, you get to "cancel out" another risk factor for heart disease (even a high total cholesterol, within reason).

Table 14.2 HDL Cholesterol Levels

Desirable	35mg/dl or higher
Low (undesirable)	34mg/dl or lower

You could think of LDL cholesterol as your *least desirable level*. The higher your LDL, the greater your risk of heart disease.

Table 14.3   LDL Cholesterol Levels

Desirable	129mg/dl or lower
Borderline high	130–159mg/dl
High	160mg/dl or higher

Other risk factors come into play when your doctor attaches significance to your cholesterol levels. A borderline high LDL might be acceptable if you have no other risk factors for heart disease (though you still want to try to bring it down through diet and exercise). If you smoke and both your parents died of heart disease at relatively early ages, your LDL just crossed the border into dangerously high. Your doctor may prescribe medication (in addition to diet and exercise) to help bring your LDL level down.

What Is Cholesterol, Anyway, and What Does It Do?

For as many problems as too much cholesterol causes, you can't live without a certain amount of the fatty substance. Chemically speaking, cholesterol is a chemical called a *lipid*. Your body uses cholesterol to make cell membranes and some hormones. Like fat, cholesterol exists in several forms. Each plays a slightly different role in how your body functions. "Good" cholesterol, or HDL, actually seems to protect your arteries from plaque buildup. "Bad" cholesterol, or LDL, accelerates plaque buildup. Scientists don't fully understand how this happens, but the correlation is unmistakable.

HDL: The "Good" Cholesterol

Not all cholesterol is bad. We often call HDL the "good" cholesterol, because it carries cholesterol back to the liver. The liver then breaks cholesterol down into waste products your body can eliminate. There's some evidence that high HDL levels also draw cholesterol from arterial plaque that has already accumulated

Cardio Care
Does a drink a day really keep LDL at bay? Some research suggests that moderate daily alcohol consumption (one to two drinks) lowers LDL and raises HDL. If you already drink a glass of wine or beer several days a week and this creates no other problems for you, fine. But don't start drinking to protect your heart. Diet and exercise also lower LDL, without the potential negative effects of alcohol use.

Just for YOU
Need another reason to give up smoking? Cigarette smoking lowers your levels of HDL, or "good" cholesterol. A lower HDL level increases your risk for heart disease.

in your arteries. HDL makes up 25 to 35 percent of your blood cholesterol. The higher your HDL, the lower your risk of heart attack. Reducing the fat in your diet and increasing your level of physical activity are lifestyle changes that raise your HDL.

LDL: The "Bad" Cholesterol

LDL is nasty stuff that sticks to the walls of your arteries. Unfortunately, you usually have more of it than HDL. The higher your LDL level, the more likely your arteries are to have fatty deposits lining their walls. Over time, these deposits can build to block the flow of blood. Like stones in a stream, they cause turbulence. This allows blood clots to form that will plug your artery either at that point or when the clots break away and flow into a narrower channel. The main goal of a low-fat diet is to lower your LDL levels to reduce this buildup.

Cardio Care

If you're taking an antioxidant supplement, check the label to see what's in it. Vitamin E is emerging as an effective tool in holding off heart disease in people who have a family history of heart problems. The health benefits of vitamin A (often in the form of beta carotene) are less clear. Too much vitamin A can poison your liver and cause birth defects. There are also unanswered questions about beta carotene's role in heart disease. If it's vitamin E you want, take a supplement that contains just vitamin E.

Lp(a): The Other "Bad" Cholesterol

As if your dietary habits weren't enough to get you into trouble with your heart, your genes have to jump in to complicate things. Between 20 and 30 percent of adults have a "special" form of LDL called lipoprotein(a), or Lp(a) for short. Lp(a) interferes with your body's ability to dissolve clots. Unfortunately, diet, exercise, and even medication seem to have little effect on lowering Lp(a). Don't give up these efforts, though. Lp(a) is only one piece of a complex process. Remember, you can't totally eliminate your risks for heart disease. You can only reduce those within your ability to control. Researchers continue to study Lp(a) and other lipids to try to understand exactly what roles they play in health and in heart disease.

Triglycerides: Another Kind of Cholesterol

Triglycerides are another form of fat closely related to cholesterol. Since what you've recently eaten influences your triglyceride level, the laboratory will draw your blood after an overnight fast (no food or drink except water).

Table 14.4   Triglyceride Levels

Desirable	199mg/dl or lower
Borderline high	200–399mg/dl
High	400–1,000mg/dl
Very high	higher than 1,000mg/dl

Familial Hyperlipidemia: A Family "Gift" You Don't Want

Sometimes high cholesterol and triglyceride levels are genetic (run in your family), a condition called *familial hyperlipidemia*. Most forms of familial hyperlipidemia respond to aggressive lifestyle changes (very low-fat diet and daily exercise) in combination with cholesterol-lowering drugs. In rare situations, the genetic influence is so strong that efforts to reduce LDL and trigylceride levels have little success. Familial hyperlipidemia is a significant risk factor for heart disease and heart attack.

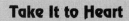

Take It to Heart

Is it just another fish story, or can eating more fish really lower your triglycerides? Though the evidence is far from conclusive, some studies suggest just that. Fish contain special polyunsaturated fats called *omega-3 fatty acids* that keep triglycerides from forming. The relationship between fish consumption and lower LDL levels has less to do with fish than with lowering overall intake of saturated fats, which happens when fish replaces red meat and other animal fats in your diet. The jury's still out on whether fish-oil supplements have the same effect, however. Your best bet for lowering triglyceride and cholesterol levels is still to reduce fat in your diet and exercise regularly.

The "Step" Diets

So you need to lower your cholesterol levels? There's a "step" diet to help you along! Step I and Step II are the same, except for fat and cholesterol intake. Your doctor may suggest the Step I diet, which is really just a plan for heart-healthy eating, to help you make a modest reduction in your blood cholesterol levels. If your total and LDL cholesterol levels are high, or if you've had a heart attack or stroke, your doctor may recommend the Step II diet, which further restricts saturated fat and cholesterol intake. The levels in both Step diets are recommended by the American Heart Association and the National Institutes of Health.

Table 14.5 Both Step Diets (Daily Levels)

Calories to maintain your desired weight	
Total fat	30% or less
Carbohydrate	55% or more
Protein	15% or so

continues

Table 14.5 Continued

Calories to maintain your desired weight	
Step I Diet	
Saturated fat	8–10%
Cholesterol	300mg or less
Step II Diet	
Saturated fat	7% or less
Cholesterol	200mg or less

Medications to Reduce Cholesterol Levels

Several medications are now available to help lower blood cholesterol levels. Cholesterol-lowering drugs work on the liver and bile-producing hormones to interfere with your body's cholesterol-making process. Don't think you can just take a pill and forget about diet and exercise, though. Like all medications, cholesterol-lowering drugs can have side effects. Except for the few people whose genes give them extraordinarily high LDL, these drugs provide a short-term boost while you get your heart-healthy lifestyle in order. Cholesterol-lowering drugs can drop your LDL 10 to 40 percent, while a low-fat diet can drop it 10 to 30 percent. If a 20-percent decrease would get your cholesterol to a desirable level, your doctor might try diet changes alone first.

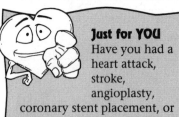

Just for YOU
Have you had a heart attack, stroke, angioplasty, coronary stent placement, or coronary-bypass graft? Your doctor might use cholesterol-lowering medication combined with a very low-fat diet to get (and keep) your LDL level below 100mg/dl. Some studies show that very low LDL levels hold off the redeposits of fatty material that cause your arteries to clog again.

Get Moving!

Regular exercise can double the rate at which your body lowers LDL after you change your eating habits. Since we've dedicated the chapters in Part 4, "Exercise Makes the Heart Grow Stronger," to physical activity, we won't say a lot here—except get moving! Use that time that's not long enough for anything else to walk around the block... or your desk. Weed the garden. Mow the lawn (but not with a riding lawn mower!). Hit a bucket of balls. Walk the dog. Shoot hoops. Play catch with the kids. Dust off your bicycle, strap on a helmet, and reconnect with your inner child (watch for traffic!). You get the picture.

What Women Need to Know: Estrogen and Cholesterol

Thanks to estrogen, women generally have lower LDL and higher HDL levels than men—until menopause. If you're a woman on the other side of menopause, you've probably considered estrogen-replacement therapy. Many factors go into making your decision. One more to consider is the beneficial effect estrogen has on cholesterol levels. Estrogen raises HDL and lowers LDL in women after menopause. Estrogen also seems to be one of the rare substances that lowers Lp(a), a particularly dangerous form of cholesterol.

Cardio Care
While reducing the fat and cholesterol in your diet is a great first step, adding exercise to the mix gives your efforts a big boost. Regular exercise raises HDL and, in some people, also lowers LDL. The combination often results in weight loss as well, which further reduces LDL levels.

"So What Should I Eat?"

In reality, eating is more than just the process of nourishing your physical body. Meals are social events, times when we enjoy the company of friends and family. And being the complicated creatures that we are, we often eat for reasons not related to nourishment—we eat to celebrate, to mourn, to relieve stress, or because sights and smells entice us to eat. You don't have to give up all your favorites to eat a more heart-healthy diet, though you might have to eat less of them, and less often. As you do, you'll cultivate new favorites that are lower in fat and cholesterol. Read product labels carefully, so you can make informed choices.

The American Heart Association recommends that you limit your average daily dietary cholesterol to no more than 300mg. Don't panic if Wednesday's level shoots over this; just adjust your intake for the day or two following. When you're looking at fat calories, remember that they, too, represent an average, not an absolute. Some foods will be higher and others lower than the recommended fat percentages. As much as possible, choose foods labeled low-fat or foods naturally low in fat (like fruits and vegetables). If you can look back at the end of the week and see that overall you stayed within the guidelines, you're doing OK. Do you know how much cholesterol your favorite foods contain? Here's a list of some common foods and their cholesterol amounts.

Table 14.6 Cholesterol Content of Common Foods

Food	Cholesterol	Saturated Fat	Total Fat
Top sirloin steak, 3 oz., broiled	77mg	5.3g	13.3g
Corned beef, 3 oz.	83mg	6.3g	16.1g
Ground beef, extra lean, 3 oz., broiled	71mg	6.2g	13.9g
Ground beef, lean, 3 oz., broiled	74mg	7.0g	15.7g

continues

Table 14.6 Cholesterol Content of Common Foods

Food	Cholesterol	Saturated Fat	Total Fat
Leg of lamb, 3 oz., roasted	79mg	5.1g	12.4g
Boneless cured ham, extra lean, 3 oz.	45mg	1.7g	4.7g
Chitterlings, 3 oz., simmered	122mg	9.2g	24.4g
Veal cutlet, 3 oz., breaded, pan-fried	95mg	3.1g	7.8g
Skinless chicken breast, half (3 oz.)	72mg	1.2g	3.0g
Ground turkey, 3 oz.	87mg	2.9g	11.2g
Smoked pork sausage link, 4 inches	37mg	6.8g	17.4g
Turkey roll, 2 slices (2 oz.), light meat	23mg	1.4g	4.0g
Cod, 3 oz., broiled	47mg	0.1g	0.7g
Atlantic salmon, 3 oz., broiled	60mg	1.1g	6.9g
Sockeye salmon, 3 oz., broiled	74mg	1.6g	9.3g
Milk (1 cup), skim	4mg	0.3g	0.4g
Milk (1 cup), 1%	10mg	1.6g	2.6g
Milk (1 cup), 2%	18mg	2.9g	4.7g
Milk (1 cup), 3.3% (whole)	33mg	5.1g	8.2g
American processed cheese, 1 oz.	27mg	5.6g	8.9g
Cheddar cheese, 1 oz.	30mg	6.0g	10.1g
Egg, whole	213mg	1.6g	5.0g
Egg white	0mg	0.0g	0.0g
Butter	28mg	6.8g	10.6g

The National Institutes of Health—National Heart, Lung, and Blood Institute.

The Least You Need to Know

➤ Not all cholesterol is bad. Your body needs cholesterol to function. Higher HDL cholesterol levels seem to protect against heart disease.

➤ Diet combined with regular physical activity is the most powerful lifestyle change for influencing cholesterol levels.

➤ Saturated fats (mostly from animal products like meat and eggs) have the greatest effect on your cholesterol level.

➤ Women who take estrogen after menopause have higher HDL and lower LDL levels than women who don't.

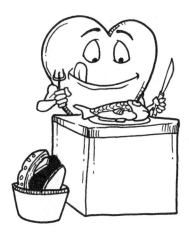

An Ounce of Prevention Is a Pound of Cure

The best way to keep your body's fat levels low is to keep your diet's fat levels low. Though not always as easy as it sounds (especially if you have a lifetime of high-fat habits to overcome), it's not an impossible mission. Do you think of heart-healthy eating as giving up all you enjoy about food? Then read on. Heart-healthy living is about making choices, not sacrifices.

How Do You Feel About Food?: A Self-Quiz

Most of us eat for a variety of reasons not related to whether we're hungry or our bodies need an infusion of nutrients. Food makes us feel good, sometimes because we associate it with pleasant experiences and sometimes because of chemicals the food contains (like chocolate). How do you feel about food? Here's a short self-quiz to help you find out:

	Yes	No
Nothing cures the blues like eating a carton of ice cream, a bag of chips, or a box of cookies.	___	___
If I leave food on my plate, a child someplace in the world goes to bed hungry.	___	___
What I like best about the holidays is that everybody eats as much as I do.	___	___
Dinner's not over till there's no more food.	___	___
No food, no party.	___	___
I eat differently when other people are around than I do when I eat alone.	___	___
No matter what rules I set for myself about what and how much to eat, I always break them once I start eating.	___	___

If you have more "yes" than "no" answers, it's time to rethink your attitudes and feelings about eating. Food is meeting other needs for you that aren't related to nutrition.

Take It to Heart

The U.S. Department of Agriculture and the U.S. Department of Health and Human Services review and update dietary guidelines for American adults every five years. First issued in 1980, the federal government's dietary guidelines form the basis of school lunch programs and other nutritional plans such as those used in hospitals and residential care facilities.

Are You Really What You Eat?

In a word, yes. Just as surely as you can't spin straw into gold, you can't grow a healthy body from junk food. What you put into your body is what your body has to work with. Take your heart, for example. It makes do with what you give it. If that's a lot of fat and few other nutrients, after a while, your heart can't make do anymore. If you want a happy, healthy heart, you have to feed it right.

Feeding the Body/Mind

Sometimes your eating habits point to imbalances in other parts of your life. How do you handle stress? Do you go for a walk or meditate... or do you scarf a week's worth of chocolate? Food often substitutes for what exercise and stress-management techniques should handle. To soothe the soul, we feed the body. Changing your eating habits is only one part of the lifestyle changes that'll make your heart happy (and healthy). Attend to these other aspects of your being, and you give your efforts in other areas a big boost.

Changing What Tastes Good

You learn taste. Ever try a jar of baby food, just out of curiosity? Bland, nasty stuff to our adult taste buds! Yet babies gurgle excitedly when they see mom or dad spooning green goop from those little jars. Then you grow up and learn that the world is filled with strange and exotic tastes—ice cream, potato chips, chili dogs, chocolate cake. You learn to like these tastes because everybody else does.

Well, your learning curve doesn't have to stop just because you're grown up now. You can keep learning to like new tastes and textures, ones that make your heart happier. In fact, many people whose bodies experience a significant trauma (like a heart attack) find their tastes different when they recover. Doctors often attribute this to interruptions in your nervous system, but could it be your body sending you a message? After three or four weeks, new tastes become the standard, and it's the old favorites that'll taste funny. But it takes some conscious effort on your part. You might fix or order favorite foods more from habit than any desire to eat them. It's like when you move to a new house not too far from your old one. For the first few weeks, your car seems to head to the old house on its own. After a while, the new route becomes automatic. Then one day, you decide to drive by the old house, just to see what it looks like now, and the route feels strange and unfamiliar. At first, it feels odd to have a salad instead of fries. After a few weeks, you might find it hard to understand why you liked fries in the first place.

How to Stay Motivated to Eat Right

Change isn't easy. In fact, it's downright hard when everyone around you stays the same. Our culture centers around what sociologists call *instant gratification*—we want it, we get it. Now. Need cash? There's an ATM in nearly every mini-mart. It's 2:00 in the morning, and you're out of bath tissue? There's probably a grocery store within 20 minutes that's open 24 hours a day. Hungry? Hit the drive-thru. (It's open late, too.)

Red Alert!
Beware products marketed as "fat-burners" and "body-shapers"—they don't and they aren't. The only way to lose fat (and weight) is to eat less and exercise more. While it might appear that you gain and lose weight more noticeably in some parts of your body than others, this is because excess body fat tends to settle (and disappear as you lose weight) in certain patterns.

Cardio Care
Do you need vitamin supplements? Most healthy adults could get the nutrients their bodies require through wise dietary choices. Excessive amounts of some vitamins, such as vitamins A and D, can be harmful. Not all multivitamin supplements are the same, and some contain more than the recommended daily levels of certain vitamins and minerals. You might need a plain mutivitamin supplement if you are on a weight-reducing diet, are a woman of child-bearing age, or are over age 65.

When you don't have to wait, you don't have time to think about why you want something and whether getting it is a good thing. When was the last time you stopped for fast food and found a plentiful supply of apples, oranges, bananas, and juices (though more mini-marts are starting to carry fresh fruits and vegetables)? When it comes right down to it, motivation comes mostly from within. No one else can make you change. Here are a few tips to help you *want* to change:

➤ **Don't deprive yourself.** In moderation, no food has to be off-limits (unless you're allergic to it). Nothing makes you crave something more than thinking you can't have it.

➤ **Try new and varied foods.** Variety prevents boredom and helps keep you from slipping back to old eating habits (which, if you think about it, are pretty boring themselves).

➤ **Plan regular meals.** Eating at the same time helps you separate food from other activities. This makes it easier to control what and how much you eat.

➤ **Keep low-fat snacks handy and high-fat snacks out of the house.** If you want an ice cream cone, fine—but make it an effort to get one.

➤ **Choose low-fat ways to prepare former favorites that you just don't want to give up.** Oven-bake chicken instead of frying (and remove the skin first). Use extra-lean ground beef and broil it, choose low-fat cheese, and hold the mayo for cheeseburgers that even your heart can handle (every now and then, though, not every day).

Keeping a Daily Food Journal

Now that you know how you make your food choices, what does cross your lips in the course of a day? A daily food log is a revealing—and useful—way to find out. It's easy to do. Just write down what you eat and when. Add comments if you want, like where you were ("at a party") and why you ate something you didn't really want ("it was there").

Keep your log where no one else will see it, so you feel comfortable being honest with yourself about what and how much you eat. Pay particular attention to how much you eat compared to the package label's serving size. Many people eat double or triple the assumed serving size without realizing they're doing so. If you're trying to lose weight, you can estimate the calories your portion contains using label information. Take your log with you when you leave the house so you can jot down any meals or snacks you have while you're away at work, shopping, or whatever.

Here's a sample of how you could do a daily food log. If journaling is a routine part of your life, your log might read more like a diary. If not, your log might be just a list. What's important is that you're honest in what you write down. The idea is to gain insights into your eating habits, not to punish yourself for eating "wrong."

Table 15.1 Daily Food Log Example

Today is... Tuesday

Time	Food or Drink	Portion Size	Label Size Serving	Estimated Calories
6am	coffee w/2 tsp. sugar	10-oz. mug	6–8 oz.	30
	bagel w/light cream cheese	1 bagel, 3 tbsp. cream cheese	1 bagel 1 tbsp. cream cheese	290 + 90 (30/tbsp.)
9:30am	1/2 doughnut	whole doughnut	——	don't know
noon	garden salad w/bleu cheese dressing	lunch special	——	300–500?
	potato roll	one	——	300?
2pm	coffee w/2 sugars	12 oz.	——	30
	sandwich cookies	6 (pkg. of 6)	3	360 (60/cookie)

Your daily food log shows you when and what you eat. Skipping meals, especially breakfast and lunch, leads to snacking—and most snack foods are less than ideal substitutes for more nutritious selections you might make at a meal. If you find yourself hungry between meals, plan to munch on heart-healthy alternatives such as fruit (fresh or dried) and other low-fat foods. Once you can see your eating patterns, you can begin making choices that are better for your health.

How Your Loved Ones Can Help

If you're making heart-healthy lifestyle changes, encourage your significant other and family members to join you. You'll be better able to support each other, and eating the same foods is definitely cheaper than shopping for two separate menus. Notice we say "encourage," which is distinctly different from "nag." If family members resist change, don't pressure. If you're the chief cook, you might gradually shift your family's diet as you shift your own.

Just for YOU
Do you have children at home? It's never too early to start training their taste buds to enjoy heart-healthy eating. While children's growing bodies need adequate dietary fat along with other nutrients, most children today eat diets with far more fat than they need. Try whole-grain waffles (hold the butter and go light on the syrup) and tofu stir-fry—you might be surprised at how quickly they catch on.

What to Do When Someone Else Is Cooking

When someone else cooks, it's sometimes harder, but not impossible, to maintain heart-healthy eating. You're at your host's mercy when you go to dinner parties and other social events where food's a big part of the festivities. This is a special challenge during holidays, when there's food everywhere.

You don't have to be a martyr. Just choose items you know are lower in fat than other options—you've read the last few chapters, and you know what these choices are. Pass on fried foods, or take very little and fill your plate with vegetables. Take small portions, especially if your host will expect you to have seconds (or more). And relax. One meal a little higher in fat won't undo your weeks, months, or years of healthy eating. Just don't let it become a pattern! Add more exercise the following day, and cut back on fat to balance your week's intake.

What to Do When You Just Have to Have It

Sometimes those urges just get the better of you. You've got to have CHOCOLATE or CHIPS or FRENCH FRIES. So go ahead. An occasional splurge won't hurt you—as long as moderation remains your guide. Buy *one* small candy bar, bag of chips, or order of fries, and eat slowly. The longer your eating habits are heart-healthy, the less enticing these "treats" will be. Most important, don't let yourself feel guilty. It's not "bad" to have cravings, only human.

By Heart
A *nutritionist* or *dietitian* is someone who has completed a program of study in nutrition or food science. Those who meet the educational and clinical requirements and pass a national test are also registered dietitians, which they designate by placing the initials "RD" after their names.

Consulting a Nutritionist

A nutritionist has special education and training in nutritional science. This healthcare professional understands dietary requirements for healthy people as well as those whose medical conditions mean they have special needs, like diabetes and heart disease. If you've had a heart attack, you've probably already talked with a *nutritionist* or *dietitian* as part of your rehabilitation program. Many hospitals and healthcare centers offer public programs about nutrition. Your doctor can also refer you to a nutritionist. If you can't find a nutritionist, the American Dietetic Association can tell you who's in your area. For information about how to contact the ADA, see Appendix B, "Resources for a Happy, Healthy Heart."

A Sample Heart-Healthy Menu You Can Live With

The secret to changing your eating habits is to create menus with foods you like. Granted, you'll probably have to save some of your former favorites for special occasions. Here are some suggestions to get you started on heart-healthy menus of your own. Your goal is to meet your personal calorie requirements (see Chapter 12, "A Full Heart") with less than 30 percent of them from fat (and less than 10 percent from saturated fat).

Remember, spice is the variety of life! It seems that everyone who's anyone has a low-fat cookbook out. If you just want to experiment, check out your local library. Even fast-food restaurants publish the nutritional content of the foods they serve. They often print this information on menus, tray covers, and napkins. The world is a friendlier place for those who care about nutrition.

Breakfast

➤ One cup whole grain, unsweetened cereal

➤ One cup 1-percent or skim milk

➤ Seasonally available fruit—try blueberries, raspberries, blackberries, strawberries, banana slices, raisins, currants, kiwi slices; be adventurous!

➤ Whole or multigrain toast (one slice of bread) with low-fat margarine, low-fat cream cheese (for variety, try the different flavored products), or fruit spread

➤ One cup orange juice (for variety, try diluting it $2/3$ to $1/3$ with flavored seltzer)

➤ Black coffee or tea if you like (try a splash of 1-percent milk or skim instead of cream or nondairy creamer, if that's how you like your coffee)

Lunch

➤ Green or pasta salad with low-fat dressing

➤ Sandwich with low-fat (lean) meats like turkey, ham, or roast beef, on whole or multigrain bread; try condiments like mustard, horseradish, pickles, green peppers, and hot or mild peppers instead of mayonnaise

➤ Raw "finger" vegetables (carrots, radishes, cucumbers, bell peppers, cauliflower, broccoli)

➤ Fresh fruit, sorbet, or sherbet

➤ Hot or iced tea with lemon, fruit juice products

Dinner

➤ Broiled chicken, fish, lean pork, or, occasionally, lean beef

➤ Red potatoes, rice, pasta (try tomato-based rather than cream sauces), or baked potato (try low-fat plain yogurt, pepper, and chives instead of sour cream and bacon pieces)

➤ Steamed or microwaved fresh vegetables (try different herbs and seasonings to give new flavor to old standards)

➤ Whole or multigrain bread or roll (try plain or with olive oil)

➤ Green salad with low-fat dressing (try different kinds for variety)

➤ Fruit cobbler, angel-food cake with fresh berries, gingerbread, fresh berries with low-fat yogurt, melon medley (different kinds of melon served together), or, occasionally, fruit pie

➤ One cup 1-percent or skim milk

Snacks

➤ Fresh and dried fruits

➤ Sliced vegetables

➤ Low-fat or no-fat crackers

➤ Low-fat yogurt with fruit

➤ Popcorn (hold the butter and butter-flavored oils)

➤ Graham crackers

➤ Bagel with low-fat cream cheese or fruit spread

➤ Pretzels

➤ Rye crisps

Check your local bookstore for cookbooks that feature easy-to-prepare low-fat recipes. Cook when you have time, and freeze leftovers for when you don't.

Dr. DeWitt's Fast Fish and Veggies Dinner

As a special treat, here's a great microwave dish that proves doctors practice what they preach. Place fresh or frozen fish filets (not breaded) in the bottom of a microwavable cooking dish. Cook for three to four minutes on medium-high. Add sliced zucchini, bell peppers, onion, and mushrooms in a layer over the fish. Splash in a little white or red wine. Cook on medium-high until fish flakes easily. You can substitute frozen vegetables if that's what you have in the freezer, or sprinkle on some dill, basil, and oregano for a bit more zip.

As a special treat, here's a great microwave dish that proves doctors practice what they preach. Place fresh or frozen fish filets (not breaded) in the bottom of a microwavable cooking dish. Cook for three to four minutes on medium-high. Add sliced zucchini, bell peppers, onion, and mushrooms in a layer over the fish. Splash in a little white or red wine. Cook on medium-high until fish flakes easily. You can substitute frozen vegetables if that's what you have in the freezer, or sprinkle on some dill, basil, and oregano for a bit more zip.

The Least You Need to Know

➤ Heart-healthy eating is about developing new tastes, not just giving up old ones.

➤ Let a single rule guide your food choices at parties and social events: moderation.

➤ Broaden your dietary horizons by trying new foods and dishes. The more variety you bring to the table, the more likely you are to leave it satisfied.

➤ You don't have to go it alone. Consult a nutritionist for help in planning your transition to a low-fat, heart-healthy diet and lifestyle.

Part 4
Exercise Makes the Heart Grow Stronger

Changing your diet seems like a snap compared to changing your activity level, doesn't it? After all, you don't need time to change the way you eat.

There's no magic formula to get more time from each day, no two-for-one split when the conditions are right, no bonus hours for hard work. But you can look at the way you spend the time you've got, just as you looked at the foods you eat. Choosing to spend 20 minutes at lunch walking around the block instead of chatting in the cafeteria is no different than grabbing an apple instead of a candy bar. (And you're not likely to be overheard talking about the boss's bad haircut while you're hoofing it down the sidewalk.)

The chapters in this section explain why exercise is so important and help you design a daily activity plan that fits your lifestyle in terms of both time and interests. And remember—the present is the gift of right now. What are you waiting for?

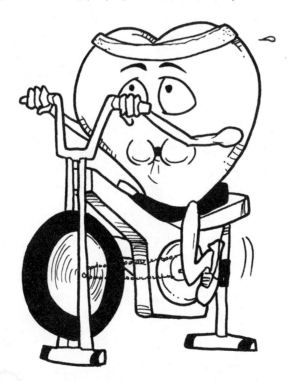

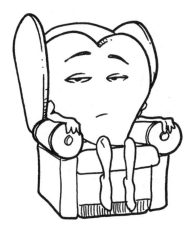

Chapter 16

Exercise, Who Needs It?

In This Chapter

➤ The drawbacks of a sedentary lifestyle

➤ How active is your day: A self-quiz

➤ Finding your fitness level

➤ Putting more activity in your life

Who needs exercise, anyway? All that sweating and heavy breathing—really, now, just who needs it? Well, check the mirror! You do. One in four Americans gets no physical exercise at all beyond the activities of daily living (sorry, no points for playing cards, even if you do jump up and down when you win). Only two in five get as much regular exercise as health experts say is necessary. What do you need? Surprisingly little—most experts recommend 20 to 60 minutes of vigorous activity at least three times a week. Recent recommendations also include lifestyle exercise such as 30 minutes of sustained activity (virtually anything from gardening to walking the dog) most days. Why the change? Most health experts realize how intimidating it is to "suit-up" and go to the gym. The new recommendations are meant to encourage most people to make exercise part of everyday life rather than a burden. So why do so few of us do it? When it comes right down to it, exercise is something you do just for you. No one else benefits as directly as you do. Yet we all find it difficult to take this time for ourselves, however brief.

What Do You Do All Day?: A Self-Quiz

Some of us have more activity in our lives than we realize, though most of us have less—and less than we need. What about you? Take this self-quiz to find out:

1. I get a 20-minute break mid-morning and mid-afternoon. I use this time to...

   A. Grab a short nap.

   B. Hey! It's a coffee break. I get a cup of coffee—and a doughnut or a candy bar.

   C. Take a short walk outside, or walk up and down a flight of stairs.

2. It's been a long day, and I'm beat. When I come home, I...

   A. Throw on some sweats and start fixing dinner.

   B. Throw on some sweats, pop a beer, and turn on the tube.

   C. Throw on some sweats, grab a flavored water, and go for a run or walk to burn off the day's stress.

3. Ah, the weekend at last! Time to...

   A. Clean the gutters, garage, or basement.

   B. Get the chips and dip ready for today's game.

   C. Go the distance at the park's fitness trail.

4. I just need a couple things from the store, and look at this! A spot right in the front. I...

   A. Circle the lot, and if the spot's still there, I figure it's got my name on it.

   B. Pull right in. What luck!

   C. Pass it up for one farther from the door, so I can get in a short walk to stretch my legs.

5. This home-fitness system is the best investment I ever made. I use it every day to...

   A. Inspire next week's exercise routine.

   B. Lay out my clothes for tomorrow.

   C. Work different muscle groups.

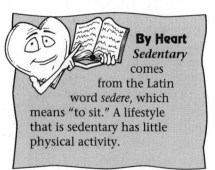

By Heart
Sedentary comes from the Latin word *sedere*, which means "to sit." A lifestyle that is sedentary has little physical activity.

If you've got a lot of Bs, you'd better be moving! Every day has dozens of opportunities to include physical activity. We tend to slide into habits that pass by those opportunities. Watch for these moments, and use them to make your heart happy. If you have mostly As, you need to close the gap between what you *should* do and what you *actually* do. And if your answers are mostly Cs, congratulate yourself for your healthy, active lifestyle.

A Sedentary Lifestyle: You Don't Want One

Ours is a *sedentary* society. We ride to work, take the elevator to the office, sit behind a desk, order lunch in, talk to each other over the phone or computer, and stop for dinner on the way home. (Not all of us, of course, but far more than ever before.) Relaxing means crashing on the couch in front of the TV until it's time to go to bed. The techno-tarpits that dot the landscapes of our lives are killing us off just as surely as the real things claimed the dinosaurs. America's fastest growing health problem is not AIDS, or cancer, or even heart disease. It's inactivity.

You Won't Live to Be 100 by Just Sitting Around

No age group in America is growing faster than the 85+'ers. While the total United States population expanded by just under 40 percent in the 30 years between 1960 and 1990, the over-85 group surged by nearly six times that rate. By the year 2040, there'll be as many as four million Americans over age 85. Scientists credit a combination of hearty genes and healthy living for the trend.

Those who hit 100 don't get there by waiting for this milestone to arrive. They've been active all their lives, many through physically demanding jobs. Moderation defines their dietary habits. They walk, do housework, garden, shop. Though the risk of dying increases dramatically in each decade after 50, it seems to slow in the 80 and 90s and beyond. Evidence, perhaps, that if you make it that far, you've earned a little reprieve. And you're never too old to add physical activity to your life. Many studies support the beneficial effects for people of all ages, from improved physical fitness to sharpened mental well-being. Activity well could be the elusive fountain of youth!

Set Small Goals You Can Reach

If you run a marathon every year, congratulations! You're no doubt in excellent shape physically, because it takes steady, consistent effort to have a body that can go the distance. Whether you aspire to run a marathon or to walk around the block, the first

Red Alert!
As important as exercise is to heart health and overall fitness, don't just leap into a program. If you are over age 50, have a condition that requires ongoing medical care, are more than 30 percent overweight, or haven't been physically active for several years, start your return to fitness with a physical exam from your doctor.

Just for YOU
Are you a woman past menopause? Osteoporosis is a particular risk for you. Once your ovaries stop producing estrogen, your bones begin to thin and become brittle. This makes them vulnerable to fractures (broken bones). Hormone replacement therapy and calcium intake help slow this process. But they can't do it all alone. Regular, vigorous exercise is the third part of the equation to slow osteoporosis.

steps are the same. Set small goals. You can't overcome decades of inactivity in a week or even a month. If exercise is a new experience for you, start slow. Walk as far as you can get in five minutes, then turn around and come back. Do it every day if you can, at least five days a week. Every two days, add two minutes until you can walk 20 or 30 minutes out (40 to 60 minutes total). Increase your pace as you grow stronger. You should see steady improvement. Keep nudging yourself to move faster and farther.

Moderate Activities (30 minutes)

Wash floors and windows

Wash and wax your car

Rake leaves

Garden

Mow the lawn (not with a riding mower!)

Push a stroller

Walk (1$\frac{1}{2}$ miles)

Swim

Bicycle (8–10mph)

Moving Toward a More Active Lifestyle

Cardio Care Whatever activities you choose, start and end with a short stretching routine. Most exercise books and videos include instructions for how to "warm-up" and "cool-down" to be sure your body's ready. "Cold" muscles are often tight, making them vulnerable to injury. Warm-up stretches gently prepare your muscles for increased activity. Cool-down stretches ease them back to their normal state.

Once you get going, add some variety. Do you usually jog? Helmet up and ride your bike—you'll be amazed at how different the same scenery looks. Join an aerobics class. Take up line dancing or ballroom dancing. Jump rope. Go ice skating or in-line skating. (Fitness experts call this cross training.) And if exercise has been a casual or on-again, off-again part of your life, give it more structure and priority. Write your activities on your calendar, both as a reminder and to formalize your commitment to yourself.

Your body has become comfortable in a lifestyle with few demands and may protest your efforts to change that. And remember, pain is *not* gain. Pain is a message from your body that something's not right. Pay attention! More often than not, you've started off doing too much too fast. Most exercise-related injuries involve strains and sprains from overdoing it. Back off a bit and see if that helps. Whatever your activities and goals, you should feel better when you exercise (even if you're tired and maybe a little sore at first), not worse. If pain continues, have your doctor check it out.

Heart-Healthy Activity for Everyone

No matter what your present level of physical fitness, activity is good for your heart (not to mention the rest of you). Walking and swimming are activities nearly everyone can enjoy. Walking is easy because it's a normal activity for most people, anyway. Walking for fitness is a bit more vigorous than strolling around the park, though. Swimming is especially good if you have a physical disability, or while you're building strength and endurance. It's no-impact, so there's little chance of hurting your feet or knees. Because the water "takes the load off," swimming lets you move more freely. Like walking, swimming can be leisurely or aerobic. Sports-oriented activities are good, too, if they interest you and you can do them. Golf, tennis, and basketball offer a fairly sustained level of activity.

Don't have time for 30 to 45 minutes of exercise at a time? Break it up into smaller chunks your schedule can handle—10, 15 minutes at a time of moderately vigorous exercise several times a day has the same beneficial effects. Do you walk on a treadmill or ride an exercise bicycle indoors? Listen to books on tape or music, read, or watch the news on television at the same time. Your computer's not the only form of intelligence that can multitask! You really have no excuse not to get active.

Cardio Care
Your body needs plenty of water when you exercise. Start your warm-up and end your cool-down routines with a glass of water. Warm or hot days pull more water from your body as sweat, so drink during exercise, too.

"Do I Have to Go to a Fitness Club?"

You certainly don't need a fitness club to get fit, though you might like the more organized environment. Fitness clubs let you try a variety of activities, work with a trainer to develop a personal fitness plan, and enjoy the company of others who have similar fitness interests. Many people like to add weight training to their regular fitness program to tone and strengthen muscles. Fitness clubs generally have state-of-the-art weight machines (and trained staff to help you build buffness without hurting yourself). You can certainly do all these things without a fitness club, too. There are dozens of excellent books and videos that show you how to do exercises properly, so you don't get hurt and you get the most benefit from them. The market for home-fitness equipment is enormous—just check any garage sale!

One drawback to going it alone is that it's easier to give up. Sharing your exercise experiences, just like sharing other activities, often makes them more satisfying. Whether you join a fitness club or exercise on your own, follow these three simple rules to get the most from your efforts:

➤ Start gradually, and give your body time to rest between activities.

➤ If it hurts, don't do it.

➤ Do what you like, and have fun.

"What's a 'Fitness Level' and Do I Have One?"

Cardio Care
Sore feet won't take you very far in any exercise. Don't skimp on good shoes. Your feet swell somewhat as the day goes on, so go shoe shopping late in the afternoon or early evening. General-purpose shoes don't cut it when it comes to physical activities. If you walk, buy walking shoes. If you jog, buy running shoes.

Red Alert!
Add weight training to your exercise program with caution! You're much more likely to hurt yourself lifting weights. Consider joining a fitness club that offers supervised weight-training programs. And if you have angina or have had a heart attack, talk with your doctor before doing any weight training. Lifting heavy weights puts a significant strain on your heart.

Even an armchair athlete has a fitness level. Exercise specialists generally assign you a classification according to how quickly you can walk a mile (and still talk when you finish). To find yours, mark out a route you know is one mile long. Many public parks have measured trails. You can also use a *pedometer* (a device you wear on your ankle that tells you how far and fast you move on foot). Time yourself with a stopwatch or a watch with a second hand (or a pedometer that has a timer). Walk as fast as you can and still feel comfortable. Don't run. You should be able to breathe without gasping. People who exercise regularly can walk a mile in about 12 minutes—a fitness level of "excellent." If it takes you longer than 17 minutes, your fitness level is "poor."

It's useful to know your fitness level when you begin an exercise program, so you know what's realistic for your state of physical fitness. You might want to check your fitness level after you've been exercising for a few weeks to measure your progress.

"I'm No Kid Anymore!"

Funny thing about these bodies of ours. As they get older, they start to betray us. Things we could do at 25 we can barely dream about at 55. Go with the flow! Chances are, there are many things that don't appeal to you anymore. Change is a normal part of life. Choose activities that you like—and that like you. You may find that your knees and ankles no longer appreciate high impact activities like running, no matter how much your heart does. But your heart's pretty flexible, and it'll be just as happy with lower-impact activities that give it the same level of workout. Try race-walking or bicycling instead of running. And add strength training to your regimen. Working your muscles against the resistance of weights (free or machine) or bands builds more muscle tissue and increases bone density, too.

Making the Most of Every Minute

What're you doing right now? Sitting, no doubt! Put this book down and stand up, nice and straight. (Wait—read this section first so you know what to do.) Lift your arms out from your sides, elbows straight and palms down, until they reach shoulder height. Hold them there for five seconds. Raise them the rest of the way over your head and touch your palms together. Hold for five seconds. Now reverse—down to your shoulders, hold, down the rest of the way. That took you, what, 15 seconds? See how easy it is to do something physical when you haven't got a minute to spare? If you have a minute, you can repeat this little activity three or four times—or add a calf raise or two to get your whole body involved. Unless it's really warm where you are, you're not even sweating. Yet don't you feel a little invigorated, a little refreshed, a little more awake?

There are dozens of pick-me-ups that you can do anywhere, anytime—shoulder shrugs, head rolls, and sitting leg raises, to name a few. Of course, these tidbits aren't nearly enough to keep your body fit and your heart healthy. But they get you moving, and that's an important first step. Take a look at your day. What opportunities does it offer for you to get in a few exercise tidbits? Anywhere you have "fidget" time, you have room for some physical activity.

Make a list of five activities you like to do that fit your lifestyle. Then pick one and start doing it *today*, while it's fresh in your mind!

Table 16.1 What Do You Like to Do?

Activity	When I Could Do It
Example: Walking	20 minutes at lunchtime
1.	
2.	
3.	
4.	
5.	

The Least You Need to Know

➤ A little bit of exercise goes a long way… and more goes even further.

➤ Let your body guide the intensity of your activities. If it hurts, don't do it.

➤ Aim for 30 minutes of moderate activity on most days (at once or cumulatively).

➤ Choose activities that you enjoy.

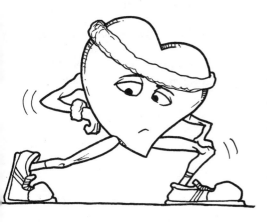

Your Transparent Heart

By now, you might know more about your heart, beating strong and steady within your chest, than other parts of your body that you see and touch every day. You should feel pretty close to this miraculous pump that gives you life.

Remember Mikhail Baryshnikov and *HeartBeat: MB*? The legendary dancer choreographed his relationship with his heart for all the world to see and share. The "music" of his beating heart, amplified for the audience to hear, is the only accompaniment Baryshnikov uses as he dances. The rhythmic beating connects body, heart, and soul. It's a performance that puts him in touch with his own mortality, the over-50 Baryshnikov says.

But being on intimate terms with your heart isn't just about mortality, about the inevitability of its demise (and yours). It's about vitality, too, the zest for life that makes living worthwhile. It's this vitality that makes *HeartBeat: MB* a personal experience for those who watch as well as he who dances. *You* dance with your heart every day. And you decide what kind of partner you want to be.

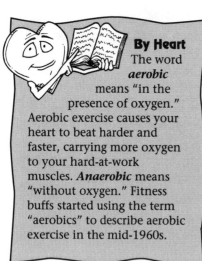

By Heart
The word *aerobic* means "in the presence of oxygen." Aerobic exercise causes your heart to beat harder and faster, carrying more oxygen to your hard-at-work muscles. *Anaerobic* means "without oxygen." Fitness buffs started using the term "aerobics" to describe aerobic exercise in the mid-1960s.

Aerobics and Your Heart

We've no doubt said it more than you care to hear: Move it! Shake those sedentary habits! Get your body in motion, no matter what you do, no matter how little time you have. Walk circles around your kitchen or desk, take the stairs (twice, just for good measure), play catch with the kids or grandkids. Doesn't sound too hard, does it? It's not. In fact, while casual activity is an excellent foundation, it's not "hard" enough, by itself, to keep your heart happy and healthy for the long haul.

Any movement is better than no movement—don't get us wrong. But to get and stay in peak form, your heart needs a good workout three or four times a week. You don't sculpt buff biceps by lifting pencils. You lift weights to create resistance, giving your biceps a reason to pull hard and firm up. Why should your heart work harder than it has to? Like your biceps, it won't without a good reason. So you've got to give it one, so it'll pump harder and faster. Weights push your biceps; *aerobic* exercise invigorates your heart.

Cardio Care
Exercise improves most chronic medical problems, from emphysema to heart failure, fibromyalgia to depression. Exercise is especially beneficial for seniors, helping to improve balance and agility as well as lower the risk of osteoporosis. This translates into less risk of falls and broken bones.

Aerobic exercise is a combination of activity, intensity, and time. When you're engaged in aerobic exercise, your muscles are using oxygen just as fast as your blood can deliver it. This helps your body release energy, as glycogen (a starch) and sugar, from fat. These substances nourish your muscles, allowing them to continue the activity for a sustained period of time. Anaerobic exercise, like lifting heavy weights, is brief and intense. It leaves waste materials, like lactic acid, in your muscles, which causes them to fatigue.

What's All That Jumping Around?

If you've ever walked past an aerobics class, it might look more like fun than exercise. Appearances are deceiving! It's fun, all right, and it's also a great workout for your body and your heart. Aerobic exercises typically work large muscle groups—buttocks and legs—for maximum conditioning. Music sets the pace and maintains the intensity level (and keeps you interested).

Table 17.1 Different Aerobics for Different Results

Kind of Aerobics	What's Involved	What It Does for You
High impact	Lots of jumping and running movements that require strong ankles and knees, as well as good balance and agility. Generally a fast pace.	High intensity for faster conditioning and fat-burning. Generally shorter sessions (20–30 minutes).
Step	Variation of high impact. Uses a 4–6-inch step or platform to step up and down. May keep you on your toes if the pace is fast.	High intensity for a vigorous workout. Can be moderate or fast.
Low impact	Movements are more fluid with less vigorous impact of your feet on the ground.	Takes longer to reach your target heart rate. Longer sessions to achieve conditioning (30–45 minutes).
Aerobic dance	Movements are more like choreographed dance steps. Can be Jazzercise or hip-hop, or anything between.	Takes longer to reach target heart rate. More artistic, may be more relaxing overall.

Exercise and Your Heart Rate

As you sit reading this book, your heart rate's probably somewhere around 70 beats per minute, give or take a few. That's typical for a resting heart rate. During aerobic exercise, you need to get your heart pounding. Did you calculate your target heart rate in Chapter 3, "Keeping Pace"? If not, go back and do it now (it's quick and easy). Remember how to take your pulse in your neck or wrist?

My target heart rate is: _____

You start conditioning your heart when your exercise pushes it to your target heart rate and keeps it there for 20 to 45 minutes at a time. Anything less, while still good for your heart, doesn't produce the same conditioning effect. (Just as lifting a pencil won't build buff biceps.)

Just for YOU
Are you less steady on your feet than you once were? Audit an aerobics class before joining. Is there a wide range of ages? Does the instructor choose movements everyone can handle with ease? Step aerobics can be especially risky if the pace is too fast for your balance and agility. Choose a class and an instructor that seem matched to your interests and physical capabilities.

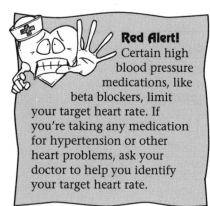

Red Alert!
Certain high blood pressure medications, like beta blockers, limit your target heart rate. If you're taking any medication for hypertension or other heart problems, ask your doctor to help you identify your target heart rate.

Red Alert!
Pay attention to pain that could be heart-related. If you experience heaviness, pressure, or pain in your chest or shoulder, stop what you're doing. Rest for a few minutes. If the pain lasts more than 15 minutes, give your doctor a call. It could be nothing—or it could be a heart attack.

No Pain, Supreme Gain

Remember that old saying, "no pain, no gain"? Throw it out the window (right behind those all-purpose sneakers you bought on sale 10 years ago)! No pain *is* gain; no pain is your goal. Pain is a direct, unmistakable message from your body to stop whatever you're doing, NOW. Pain means something's injured. You'll keep getting those jabs from angry nerves until the wound heals, whether it's a strain, sprain, cut, or bruise. So listen up, and back off. Your body will let you know when it's OK again to use your foot or knee or quadriceps (thigh muscles) or whatever it is that hurts.

Don't confuse minor aches and soreness with genuine pain, though. It's normal for your body to feel the effects of your new exercise efforts, especially if it's been living the life of leisure. How do you know which it is? Generally speaking, pain affects just one location (ankle, knee, wrist), while aches and soreness affect a group of muscles (legs, back, arms). Aches and soreness often feel better with gentle stretching and don't usually keep you from doing the activity that caused them. Whatever you call it—pain, ache, stiffness, soreness, owee—don't ignore it. If your feet feel sore after yesterday's three-mile walk, do something different today. Go for a swim or ride a bike. Or rest, which is an important part of your exercise cycle.

Starting an Everyday Heart-Healthy Exercise Program

So how do you get started? If it's been a *really* long time since you've done anything physical, wander through a fitness club to see what's available (most will give you a visitor's pass for one free visit). What did you enjoy when you were active? Tackle football's probably out of the question by now, though basketball, tennis, racquetball, volleyball, squash, swimming, running, and bicycling (whew!) are likely replacements. You don't have to stay with your first choice, or with any choice. In fact, variety is the *best* choice to keep your interest—and your participation—high.

Consider joining that fitness club you toured or hiring a personal trainer. It's fun and motivating to share your exercise time with others. And you'll learn how to do a wide variety of exercises—aerobic, endurance, and strengthening—to give your body a full workout. Whether you seek guidance or go it alone, be sure your program includes these essential elements:

➤ **The right stuff.** Would you jog in a suit? Not unless it's made of fleece or rip-stop nylon. Dress shoes? Only if they're sneakers. Don't blow your paycheck at the local sports superstore. But do invest in the right gear for your chosen activities, starting from the ground up. Buy aerobics shoes if you're doing aerobics, basketball shoes if you're playing basketball, running shoes for jogging, walking shoes for walking—you get the picture. Wear comfortable clothes. Some sports have special clothing—padded shorts are great to protect delicate body parts from hard bicycle saddles, and body-hugging leotards stay out of the way when you're doing aerobics. But sweats or shorts and a T-shirt often work just fine. Go for comfort!

➤ **Warm up and cool down.** Use gentle stretching movements to loosen your muscles before exercising and to ease them back to normal activity afterward. This allows your muscles to work efficiently and helps prevent injuries.

➤ **Variety.** Mix it up to keep yourself interested as well as to work different muscle groups for overall fitness.

➤ **Rest.** Exercise is more a cycle than a program. Your body needs to recover from its workout so it can convert all that energy to productive use. All work and no rest wears your body—and your spirit—down.

➤ **Fun.** Life's too short for tight shoes and burnt toast. Enjoy what you do! If aerobic dance doesn't turn your crank, try swimming or bicycling. Pick what you like to do, and exercise will be something you escape *to*, not *from*.

Ask Your Doctor

How long has it been since you've done anything more athletic than tying your tennis shoes? Your exercise program should start with a checkup from your doctor if

➤ You're a man over 40 or a woman over 50.

➤ You're more than 30 percent overweight.

➤ You have high blood pressure, heart disease, diabetes, or any other health condition for which you receive regular medical care.

➤ Heart disease or stroke runs in your family.

➤ You haven't had a physical exam for three or more years.

If physical activity has been part of your life for as long as you can remember (or three years, whichever is greater), wonderful! Your fitness level is probably good. Even so, it wouldn't hurt to check with your doctor before intensifying your workouts.

When?

People debate about whether morning or evening is better for exercise as they do about political candidates. In the end, the result is about the same. There is no one "right" for everyone. When does your natural energy level peak? If you rise before the sun, probably in early afternoon. If you're a night owl, probably in the evening. You might like to start your day with an exercise routine to wake yourself up or to get it in before other responsibilities steal the time. Exercise, particularly aerobic, does wake up your body. Many people like to exercise at midday to get that energy boost that will carry them through the otherwise drowsy hours that follow lunch. Intensive exercise late in the day could keep you awake longer than you want.

Experiment! Try a week of morning exercise, then a week of evening exercise. Which leaves you feeling refreshed and revitalized? In the end, the right time to exercise is the time that's right for you.

How Often?

You need a good aerobic workout session at least three days a week. Four days a week is better; five days a week is pushing it. Try alternating days to give your body time to rest and recover. Consistency gives your body a foundation to build on. If you're away from regular aerobic exercise for more than a week, you'll find you have to resume at a somewhat lower level of intensity and work your way back to where you were. On days you don't have an aerobic activity, try something different. Stroll through the park or on the beach and enjoy the sights, sounds, and smells that surround you.

How Long?

Your heart needs to beat at its target rate for 30 to 45 minutes to gain conditioning benefits from aerobic exercise. Because aerobic activities continuously feed your muscles, once your body's in shape, this seems like no time at all. Even if you feel like you could run all day, don't. Fitness experts recommend that you limit aerobic activity to no more than an hour at a time to give your body a chance to recover.

Take It to Heart

Not so long ago, "fitness" meant "calisthenics"—vigorous activities like pushups, situps, chin-ups, squat thrusts, jumping jacks, and running. But exercise isn't just for kids and military recruits. Fitness is for everyone. While old-fashioned calisthenics are fine if your physical condition permits you to do them, activities like walking and swimming can give you the same benefits.

> ### Take It to Heart
>
> Today, fitness is an industry that generates several billion dollars in annual sales of specialized clothing, footwear, equipment, and club memberships. Yet we still find comfort in the familiar. The top-selling home-fitness machine is the treadmill, which lets us walk miles without ever leaving the living room.

What About Goals?

There are basically two kinds of goals: today and tomorrow. What do you want to accomplish today? (Or what will today let you accomplish, if your life's busy.) These are immediate, action-oriented goals—play racquetball at lunch, jog around the track after work, bicycle to the post office. Tomorrow goals are more general and represent achievements—climb the stairs at work without huffing, run the Boston marathon, lose 20 pounds. Choose goals that matter to you.

Don't worry about whether your goals are big enough—if they're important to you, that's all that counts. And remember, no goal is carved in stone! You can change your today goals as the day changes and your tomorrow goals as you achieve them or as your interests change. Don't just drop a goal, though—replace it with another. This is especially important with today goals, because "I don't have time" is a very slippery slope. If you can't make it to the track after work, get in a quick run around the block before dinner. If you can't ride your bicycle outdoors, put in 20 or 30 minutes on a stationary cycle.

What are your personal exercise and fitness goals for today (daily or short-term) and for tomorrow (long-term)? List a few of each here while you're thinking about them. Use a pencil so you can change them as you progress.

> ### Red Alert!
> Ah, there's nothing like a sauna or soak in a hot tub to ease tired muscles. Just don't indulge right after exercising. Wait at least an hour, so your body has time to return to normal. And drink water, not alcohol, to avoid serious dehydration. You can sweat the equivalent of 2 glasses of water every 15 minutes you're in the hot tub! If you have high blood pressure or heart disease, talk to your doctor about safe ways to enjoy a little heat.

Table 17.2 Your Today and Tomorrow Goals

My Today Goals	My Tomorrow Goals
Example: Ride my bicycle 8 miles	Ride my bicycle 67 miles roundtrip to the Post Office in the Peninsula Metric Century Ride in June
1.	
2.	
3.	
4.	
5.	

Massaging Your Way to Heart Health

Massage is a wonderful (and relaxing) way to end a particularly vigorous workout. Many organized athletic events like bicycle rides and marathon races offer massage to participants. Massage after intense exercise increases blood flow to help muscles relax, preventing or relieving muscle spasms and aches. It also reduces fluid retention. Professional massage therapists undergo extensive training and are usually licensed by the state to

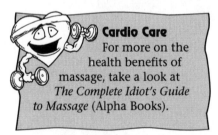

Cardio Care
For more on the health benefits of massage, take a look at *The Complete Idiot's Guide to Massage* (Alpha Books).

practice. No one to give you a massage? Try some self-massage on your lower back, neck, lower legs, and feet. Hold your fingers together and use firm (not too hard) pressure to knead the muscles in these areas.

Massage is also effective at increasing circulation and lowering blood pressure. A recent study conducted at Bowling Green State University in Ohio showed a marked decrease in systolic and diastolic blood pressure after a 15-minute chair massage.

How a Heart-Healthy Body Feels... Happy!

Notice what happens the next time you start an aerobic exercise. You might feel at first like you really don't want to do this. You're tired, nothing's going right at work, and the dirty laundry's overflowing. You start your warm-ups feeling a little grumpy, then you get underway—running, swimming, bicycling, aerobics, whatever activity you've chosen. By the time you reach your target heart rate, the bounce in your step is genuine. The boss, the kids, the bills—none of that seems to matter anymore. Your sweat carries the stress from your body. Then "it" happens. You hit brain-rush, that point where the *endorphins* (natural, feel-good chemicals your brain releases) kick in. You could go like this forever. All you hear is your heartbeat, all you feel is your muscles pushing, reaching, stretching.

We talk a lot about the physical benefits of exercise. There are so many, and many are so obvious. Muscle tone, weight loss, lower blood pressure and cholesterol, increased stamina—and of course, your ship-shape heart. Is that the glow of health that shines from your eyes? It's true—when your body feels good, it shows. Vigorous exercise gives you a natural "high," a sense of joy that you're alive. This exhilaration lasts for several hours after you've put your running shoes away. It leaves you calmer, more relaxed, more at peace with your world—at least for right now. With today's hectic lifestyles, that alone is worth your weight in gold! (Go ahead, treat yourself to a nice, crisp apple or a juicy slice of watermelon. You deserve it!)

The Least You Need to Know

➤ Aerobic exercise that pushes your heart to its target rate and keeps it there for 20 to 45 minutes is the best way to condition both your body and your heart.

➤ Pain is not a measure of success when it comes to exercise (or much else). Minor aches and soreness are common, especially as you begin your lifestyle of physical activity. Pain means you're overdoing it or you have an injury.

➤ Select exercise activities that you enjoy, and establish reasonable goals that matter to you.

➤ Exercise improves most chronic medical problems, and refreshes your spirit as it conditions your body.

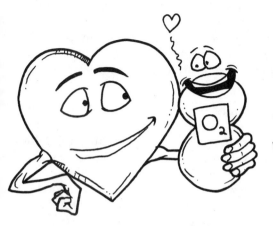

Oxygen: You Can't Live Without It

"All I need is the air that I breathe," is a refrain from a popular song from the 1970s. While other nutrients are, of course, important, nothing tops oxygen for sustaining life. You can live seven to ten days without food, three or four days without water, and three to five minutes without oxygen.

The Breath That Moves You

It seems so simple. You breathe in, you breathe out. You breathe in, you breathe out. It's a pattern that repeats itself about 15 times a minute when you're resting, up to as much as 80 times a minute during vigorous exercise. You don't have to plan it or even think about it. It just happens. Or does it?

Respiration, as doctors call this cycle, is really a complex system of chemical and neurological actions. It starts when the pressure inside your *alveoli*—the tiny balloon-like sacs deep inside your lungs where the oxygen–carbon dioxide exchange takes place—drops below the outside air pressure. This triggers the muscles of your chest, most noticeably your diaphragm, to contract. This expands your chest and initiates *inspiration*. When the pressure in your alveoli gets higher than that of the air outside, the process reverses, and *expiration* occurs. Your diaphragm and other chest muscles relax, allowing your chest to get smaller again. Of course, any system under pressure needs some sort of frame too hold all the parts in place. Your ribs, spine, collarbones, and breastbone form the frame for your lungs.

By Heart
Inspiration is the process by which your lungs take in air. It's also called *inhalation*. *Expiration* is the process of air leaving your lungs and is also called *exhalation*.

You can feel the breathing process quite easily. Sit or stand up straight. Place one hand flat against your belly and the other flat across your chest. Consciously take in a deep, slow breath. Do you feel your diaphragm rise and your chest expand? Let your breath out slowly. Do you feel your diaphragm drop and your chest relax? If you don't, don't worry. It's still taking place, even though you can't feel it. In fact, when you're breathing naturally and correctly, you can't feel your chest move very much at all, though you can feel your abdomen (diaphragm) move. Certain breathing exercises, including yoga, focus on increasing your awareness of the muscles and actions involved in breathing. You can use controlled breathing patterns to manage stress and, in chronic chest conditions, pain.

Your heart, lungs, and diaphragm work together.

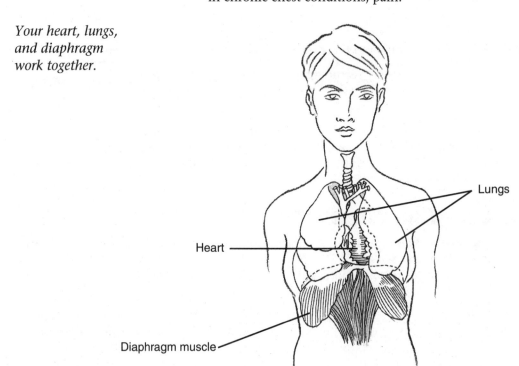

Lungs

Heart

Diaphragm muscle

Why Cardiorespiratory Fitness Is Important

You remember from Chapter 3, "Keeping Pace," that your heart and lungs work more closely together than any business partners. Without your lungs to bring in oxygen and take out carbon dioxide, your heart would have little to do… and not much time to do it in. And without your heart to send the gift of life throughout your body, your lungs would work for naught. As aerobic exercise strengthens your heart, it increases the capacity of your lungs. The deeper your chest expands, the more air your lungs can take in. And the more air your lungs take in, the more oxygen your blood carries out—a valuable aid when you're exercising.

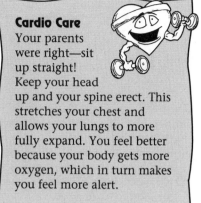

Cardio Care
Your parents were right—sit up straight! Keep your head up and your spine erect. This stretches your chest and allows your lungs to more fully expand. You feel better because your body gets more oxygen, which in turn makes you feel more alert.

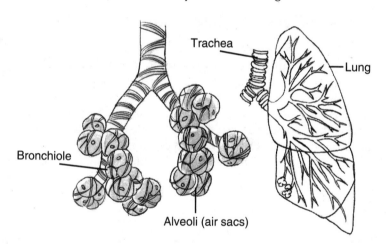

Trachea

Lung

Bronchiole

Alveoli (air sacs)

When you breathe deeply and fully, your lungs will expand. The tiny air sacs, alveoli, exchange carbon dioxide for oxygen in the blood. The deeper the breath, the more oxygen enriches the blood carried throughout your whole body. Exhale, and you release waste carbon dioxide.

Oxygen-Rich Blood

In a simplistic way, the red blood cells that carry oxygen throughout your body are like cargo cars on a train. Whether they're partially or completely loaded, they still go where the train (your bloodstream) takes them. Under normal circumstances, each red blood cell contains about 350 million molecules of a chemical substance called *hemoglobin*. Each hemoglobin molecule can hold, or bind with, four molecules of oxygen. Your red blood cells can really carry a load when they leave your lungs!

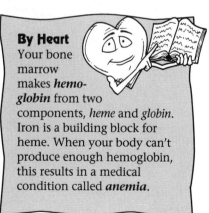

By Heart
Your bone marrow makes *hemoglobin* from two components, *heme* and *globin*. Iron is a building block for heme. When your body can't produce enough hemoglobin, this results in a medical condition called *anemia*.

Just for YOU

Are you a menstruating woman? Your monthly blood loss, particularly if it's heavy, can put you at risk for anemia. Though pregnancy gives you a break from menstruation, your developing baby draws heavily from your iron stores. Doctors recommend that pregnant women take supplements to keep their iron levels high. Your doctor can check for anemia with a simple blood test right in the office.

In some situations, your red blood cells may not carry a full complement of hemoglobin, a medical condition called *anemia*. There are many forms and causes of anemia. Blood loss and not getting enough iron from your diet cause the most common kinds of anemia. Menstruating women are at particular risk for anemia because of their monthly blood loss. A diet short on folic acid (remember those green vegetables from Chapter 12, "A Full Heart"?) or vitamin B_{12} (which comes from meat) also can cause anemia. When you have anemia, your red blood cells have less hemoglobin and can carry less oxygen. Your cells complain when they don't get enough oxygen, which your body signals to you through symptoms like headache and fatigue. Severe anemia can also cause angina if your heart doesn't get all the oxygen it needs.

The Effects of Smoking

Are you lighting up a cigarette? Then you're sending red blood cells out of your lungs without their full load of oxygen. One by-product of *combustion* (something burning) is carbon monoxide. When the fire's just outside your lips and incoming air is filled with smoke, you're flooding your lungs with carbon monoxide. (Yep, the same noxious stuff that your car's exhaust blows out.) Those pushy, selfish little carbon monoxide molecules cut right in on the oxygen molecules, binding with the hemoglobin. This leaves less oxygen for the cells that need it. The tars and residues from inhaled cigarette smoke also plug your alveoli, further interfering with your lung's efforts to get oxygen into your body. (We'll talk more about cigarette smoking and its effects on your heart and other body systems in Chapter 21, "Light Up Your Heart, Not a Cigarette.")

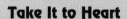

Take It to Heart

According to the principles of yoga, breathing is both the essence and measurement of life. Yoga measures the length of life not in years but in numbers of breaths. Each breath you take not only maintains your life but also extends it. The average person breathes 20,000 to 30,000 times a day, taking in about 4,000 gallons of air.

Yogis Know About Prana... Do You?

Yoga combines philosophy and physical movements to achieve a healthy balance between your body, mind, and spirit. Controlled breathing forms the basis of many yoga practices, from elementary deep breathing to more complex techniques. Your breath, according to yoga, contains essential energy called *prana*. Controlling this energy, and the power of breathing, is called *pranayama*.

Pranayama emphasizes awareness of your breathing. What's happening in your body and in your mind as you breathe? What connection exists between your state of mind and your physical condition? How does your breathing change when you're frightened... angry... excited... calm? As your body follows your mind, so your mind can follow your body. *Yogis*—people who practice yoga—use various breathing techniques to change the way their bodies and minds feel.

Breathing Lessons

"I don't need breathing lessons! Breathing's as natural as... breathing!" Of course you can already breathe, or you wouldn't be reading this book. How many different ways of breathing can you think of right now? Breathing is your body's expression of its needs, from frantic near-hyperventilation when you're frightened ("Let's get out of here!") to the slow, chest-raising pattern that signals sleep. So what's to learn? Sit up straight and pay attention!

Cardio Care
Consider taking an introductory class in yoga or breathing techniques. There, you'll learn how to pace your breathing and how to breathe deeply without hyperventilating (breathing so rapidly that too much carbon dioxide leaves your system, causing you to feel faint or dizzy). Or try an instructional videotape or book. Like other forms of fitness, you must perform breathing techniques correctly to benefit from them.

Take It to Heart

You don't have to be a yogi to use breathing techniques. Athletes know that their performance often depends on how well they can control their breathing. Divers know just when to inhale... hold... exhale. So do weightlifters, runners, bicyclists, and even dancers, among others. Most body-conditioning and toning activities incorporate controlled breathing for maximum results.

The more air you can draw into your lungs, the more oxygen that's available for your red blood cells to carry out to your body's tissues. Scientifically, this is called *tidal*

195

volume—the amount of air that moves in and out of your lungs during each respiratory cycle. A typical pair of human lungs can hold a maximum of about 4$\frac{1}{2}$ quarts, or just over a gallon, of air (4.5 liters). A typical pair of human lungs seldom fills to that level, however. At rest, most of us exchange little more than half a quart ($\frac{1}{2}$ liter) with each breathing cycle. The only time we even approach maximum capacity is during vigorous exercise when our bodies demand lots of oxygen.

Take It All In

Why does it matter if you use just a portion of your total lung capacity? Remember that the whole point of breathing is to get oxygen to your red blood cells so they can ferry it out to the body cells that need it for the activities that keep you breathing in the first place. The more efficiently your lungs and heart handle this task, the more effectively other cells can manage their tasks. Consistently low levels of oxygen, over time, cause a variety of cumulative damage, from premature tissue death to *atherosclerosis* (hardening of the arteries). So fill 'em up!

Take It to Heart

Have you ever had surgery? Breathing exercises are a routine part of your recovery and often start before you're fully awake after your operation. Hospital staff will have you cough and deep breathe, and sometimes breathe into a device called an *incentive spirometer* (where you use a tube with a small plastic ball or marker that moves as you take a deep breath in through a mouthpiece). Breathing exercises help keep fluids from settling in your lungs and also improve your state of mind by getting more oxygen (and alertness) to your brain.

Alternate Nostril Breathing

This simple yoga breathing technique is great for stress relief as well as expanding your breathing capacity. (If you have a cold or allergies that are causing congestion, try this another time when your nose is clear.) Read through the steps first, then put the book aside and give it a try. Ready?

1. Sit tall, with your spine straight and your head level (chin pointing out, not up or down).
2. Hold your right nostril closed. Breathe in, slow and deep, through your left nostril. Hold the breath in your lungs.
3. Release your right nostril and close your left nostril. Then breathe out, slow and deep, through your right nostril.

4. Alternate in and out. Hold your left nostril closed, and breathe in through your right nostril. Hold the breath in your lungs. Release your left nostril and close your right nostril. Breathe out, slow and deep, through your left nostril.

5. Repeat each pattern 10 to 12 times, three to four times a day or when you feel particularly stressed.

Do you feel stress and tension flow from your body with each repetition? Do your back, shoulder, neck, and chest muscles feel more relaxed? As long as you breathe in and out slowly and deeply, you can't overdo this exercise.

Increase Your Lung Capacity

So how do you get more from those sponge-like organs in your chest? If "aerobic exercise" is not about to roll off your tongue, go back to Chapter 17, "Your Transparent Heart," and take notes! Getting your heart pounding and your muscles working is the best way to increase your body's demand for oxygen, which in turn increases your lungs' ability to provide it. Yoga techniques are another excellent way to improve your breathing capacity and are particularly handy because you can do them just about anywhere (and you won't need a shower when you finish).

The Least You Need to Know

➤ Breathing may seem automatic, though it's really an intricate interaction among various body systems.

➤ The more air you draw into your lungs, the more oxygen your red blood cells can transport to other body tissues.

➤ Aerobic exercise and breathing techniques like those of yoga help expand your lung capacity. Not getting enough oxygen means that your body tissues can't function efficiently or effectively.

➤ Cigarette smoking reduces the amount of oxygen that enters your lungs and your bloodstream. It's the most destructive thing you can do to your lungs and heart.

out It

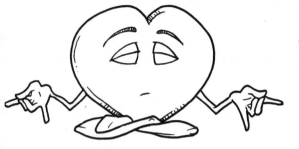

Heart-Safe Ways to Enjoy Being Active

Some people prefer to sweat solo, and some like to have company. Some activities you can do either alone or with others, like walking, jogging, and bicycling. No matter what your present fitness level and interests are, there's something to engage you.

What Do You Like to Do?: A Self-Quiz

Which physical activities you do matters less than whether you do them regularly. And if you don't like them, we can just about guarantee they'll slide off your schedule and out of your life before you finish this book. Which physical activities interest you?

1. When it comes to working up a sweat, I'd rather...

    A. Never let 'em see me.

    B. Let it all hang out with the other sweathogs.

    C. Wear dark colors so it doesn't show.

    D. Not, thanks.

2. When I was younger, I had a pretty mean...

    A. Curve ball.

    B. Hook shot.

    C. Slice.

    D. Case of road rash.

3. I've always wondered what it would be like to...

    A. Run in a marathon.

    B. Ride in one of those big bicycle events.

    C. Sink a hole in one.

    D. Spin a basketball on my finger.

4. Nothing gets my blood flowing like...

    A. A hike in the mountains.

    B. A pickup game of basketball.

    C. Bowling a perfect frame.

    D. Losing the remote control.

5. When I dream of glory, I see myself...

    A. Dancing center stage.

    B. Catching the winning touchdown pass.

    C. Setting the world record in the backstroke.

    D. Winning a lifetime free pass to the More-Than-Even-You-Can-Eat buffet.

6. My favorite part of the summer Olympics is...

    A. Track and field.

    B. Interviews with the athletes where they talk about their practice routines.

    C. Synchronized swimming.

    D. Those clever fast-food commercials.

7. I've been working really hard this week, and I need a break. I think I'll...

    A. Hit that evening aerobics class.

    B. Get in 18 holes before dark.

    C. Try a new yoga position.

    D. See a movie.

Do your answers give you a sense for whether you prefer to be with others or alone? You might like both, which certainly broadens your options. If you've marked a lot of Ds, though, your relationship with your couch is a little too cozy! Even if you've never thought of yourself as athletic, there are plenty of sports and physical activities you can try.

Engaging Your Heart in Team Sports

Team sports are a great way to combine exercise, socializing, and friendly competition all in one package. Most communities have a variety of organized team activities that target different age levels. Some teams receive support from local businesses to pay for expenses like uniforms and league fees. Others are more loosely organized and rely on members to pay for any team needs. Nearly all sports require you to buy your own personal gear. Some team sports emphasize collective ability. Others support individual effort for the common good. Still others require the participation of others, although they aren't really team sports.

Red Alert!
Temperature extremes place additional stress on your heart and other organ systems. Light activity for short periods of time is better than strenuous exercise when it's very hot or very cold outside. Remember to drink plenty of water, even in the cold when you don't think you need fluids.

Table 19.1 Team Sports—Collective Ability

Sport	Special Equipment	Aerobic Potential	Risks
Basketball	Shoes	Moderate to high	Sprains and strains
Softball	Cleated shoes, ball glove, maybe uniform, and protective gear	Low to moderate	Sprains, strains, bumps, and bruises
Volleyball	Shoes	Moderate to high	Sprains, bruises, strains
Soccer	Cleated shoes, shin guards	High	Sprains, bumps, bruises, strains

Table 19.2 Team Sports—Individual Ability

Sport	Special Equipment	Aerobic Potential	Risks
Bowling	Shoes, bowling ball	Low to moderate	Twisting injuries, sprains, strains
Swimming	Swimwear	Moderate to high	Soreness, shoulder or other, tendinitis
Shuffleboard	Cue, disks	Low	Slips or falls

Table 19.3 Multiple-Participant Sports

Sport	Special Equipment	Aerobic Potential	Risks
Golf	Cleated shoes, clubs, balls	Low to moderate	Twisting injuries
Tennis	Shoes, racquet, balls	Moderate to high	Sprains, strains, twisting injuries
Handball	Glove, shoes, balls	High	Sprains, strains, twisting injuries
Racquetball, Squash	Racquet, shoes, balls	High	Sprains, strains, twisting injuries
Table tennis	Paddles, balls	Low to moderate	Slips or falls
Sparring	Gloves, shoes, protective gear	Moderate to high	Bruises, bumps, concussions
Badminton	Racquet, shuttle-cocks (birdies)	Low to moderate	Stretching or twisting injuries

Going Solo

Sometimes you just want to get out there and push yourself or enjoy a little solitude. There are many individual sporting activities that you can do by yourself or in the company of others.

Table 19.4 Individual Sports

Sport	Special Equipment	Aerobic Potential	Risks
Walking	Shoes	Moderate	Sprains, strains, soreness
Bicycling	Bicycle, shoes, helmet, gloves, padded shorts	Moderate to high	Scrapes, sore seat, broken bones, risk of serious head injury (ALWAYS wear a helmet!)
Running	Shoes, clothing	High	Sprains, strains
Downhill skiing	Skis, boots, poles, warm clothing	Moderate	Falls (sprains, broken bones), hypothermia
Cross-country skiing	Skis, boots, poles, warm clothing	Moderate to high	Falls (sprains, broken bones), hypothermia
Horseback riding	Horse, boots, helmet, clothing, saddle, riding gear	Low to moderate	Risk of serious injury from falls

Sport	Special Equipment	Aerobic Potential	Risks
Kayaking, Canoeing	Kayak or canoe, paddles, life vest, possibly helmet	Moderate to high	Risk of drowning, hypothermia
Hiking	Correct footwear for terrain and weather, emergency kit, maps	Moderate to high	Sprains, strains, risk of getting lost
Ice skating, In-line skating	Skates, pads, helmet	Moderate to high	Sprains, strains, broken bones

A Heart for the Great Outdoors

Do you enjoy the sun and fresh air? Your body does. When your skin soaks up those rays, it's helping your bones to use vitamin D to keep them strong and sturdy. Don't overdo it, though. Too much sun is a problem for your skin. Take care to protect yourself from sunburn with a sunscreen that's at least SPF 15. You'll still get the benefits of sun exposure, with less risk of damaging your skin. Many sports and activities among those we've listed in the tables take place outdoors, combining a good workout with fresh air and sunshine. And being outside just makes you feel good! Prepare for the weather conditions, especially if you'll be out all day.

Baryshnikov Revisited

Ah, Baryshnikov. Dance personified. Such grace, such strength, such fitness. As he approached age 50, the master of ballet decided it was time try something new. He shifted his focus to modern dance because, he said, modern dance taught him how to pace and concentrate on the movements of the steps. While you might never dance like Baryshnikov, you might enjoy letting a little of the dancer in you come out. Dance comes in many forms, from boot-scootin' western line dancing to ballet-esque modern dance.

The great thing about dance is that it doesn't feel like exercise, yet it gives you a workout worthy of any aerobic activity. It also connects your mind and body through the creativity of your movements. There's less focus on strength, more on balance and flow. Just let yourself feel the music, and your body will take over from there.

Just for YOU
Where there's enough demand, community centers and fitness clubs offer wheelchair aerobics and other exercise opportunities for athletes with special needs (such as vision and hearing impairments). Activities like basketball, volleyball, and table tennis require little adaptation for wheelchair participants and can give you a good workout. Special hand-pedaled bicycles are increasingly common. And swimming lets you leave the chair behind (depending on your level of paralysis) for aerobic and strength conditioning.

> **Take It to Heart**
>
> Many world-class athletes, from football players to boxers, incorporate dance and Eastern practices like yoga and meditation into their fitness routines. These activities increase awareness, improve balance and flexibility, and help athletes focus and relax.

Yoga and Tai Chi: The Heart of the East

> **Red Alert!**
> Did you know that wind can make even moderate temperatures hazardous? Your body keeps itself warm by heating the layer of air around it. Wind removes this cushion, continually cooling your body. Even in heat, wind can be a problem. Wind causes perspiration to evaporate more quickly from your skin, which might feel good but can seriously dehydrate you if you're not drinking plenty of water.

While we recognize and sometimes even mention the overall sense of satisfaction we feel after strenuous physical activity, we don't usually look to exercise as a way to calm the mind and soothe the soul while it works the muscles. In America, we tend to view fitness as an event for the body alone. Eastern practices look at fitness differently. They often combine the physical and the philosophical, striving to balance the whole being.

To the casual observer, practices like yoga and tai chi hardly seem athletic. After all, the movements are so painstakingly slow and the positions so unusual, they can't possibly do anything for fitness. Can they? Admittedly, you won't want to replace your aerobic activities with yoga and tai chi. But if you add either or both to your overall fitness regimen, you'll soon see impressive improvements in your flexibility, balance, and breathing (aerobic capacity). The best way to learn yoga or tai chi is to enroll in a class. Like other exercises, it's important to do these correctly. Both practices require a form and degree of discipline that differs from other exercises.

Finding a Fitness Guru, Coach, Personal Trainer...

Whether you go solo or join a team, it helps to have someone on the sidelines shouting encouragement and cheering you on. Not just a loving spouse or a supportive friend, but someone who knows more about your chosen activities than you do. Most fitness clubs have qualified fitness trainers on staff to help you determine your fitness level and to plan activities to meet your fitness needs. These friendly folks typically come around while you're sweating away, offering encouragement and motivation to keep you pushing. They also make sure that you start out with warm-ups, perform your activities and exercises correctly, and finish with cool-down stretches.

You don't have to join a club to get these benefits, however. If your budget allows, you can hire a personal trainer to design a fitness program for you. A trainer should also meet with you regularly to see how you're progressing and to change your program to meet your changing needs. Before signing on with a fitness club or a trainer, talk to others who've used the same one. It's important to get a good match with your interests and needs (and sometimes age group). Here are a few tips to help you find the right match for you:

➤ **Check, don't just ask for, credentials and references.** If your prospective trainer rattles off a string of alphabet soup, ask what it all means. Check professional affiliations and certifications (the organization can usually tell you if the trainer is affiliated or has the qualifications he or she claims). How long has the trainer been in practice? Where did he or she receive training?

➤ **Observe your fitness guru in action.** Sit in on a couple different classes if the trainer works for a fitness center, or ask to come along on a meeting with a client. Many people who choose a personal trainer cherish their privacy, though you should be able to find someone willing to let you observe at least for a little while. How does the trainer keep things moving? Do participants seem to enjoy the workout? How does the trainer handle the pace of the class when someone can't keep up?

➤ **Obtain, in writing, a statement of responsibilities and commitment.** Do you have to pay for a year in advance? Exactly how much are the fees and charges, and what do they cover? What happens if things just don't work out?

➤ **Consider style.** Is your prospective trainer flamboyant and outgoing or reserved? How does this fit with your personality? Do you like a steady flow of, "C'mon, you can do it! Push! Push! You've got it! Keep it moving!" or do you prefer occasional suggestions and a pat on the back when you're done?

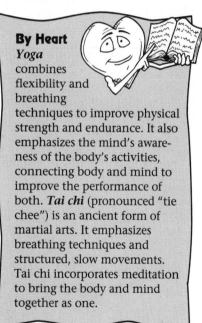

Cardio Care
It doesn't hurt to take a light jacket if you're going hiking or bicycling, just in case the weather turns sour on you. Take a whistle, so you can signal for help if you get lost or injured (it takes less energy to blow than to shout and makes more noise), and a small first-aid kit. And always carry water, even if you think you'll be back before you get thirsty.

By Heart
Yoga combines flexibility and breathing techniques to improve physical strength and endurance. It also emphasizes the mind's awareness of the body's activities, connecting body and mind to improve the performance of both. *Tai chi* (pronounced "tie chee") is an ancient form of martial arts. It emphasizes breathing techniques and structured, slow movements. Tai chi incorporates meditation to bring the body and mind together as one.

The Least You Need to Know

➤ Choosing activities you like makes it more likely that you'll do them regularly.

➤ Sports come in all levels of complexity.

➤ A qualified fitness trainer can help you get your exercise life organized.

➤ What's good for the body is good for the mind.

➤ Playing is fun and heart-healthy, too!

Part 5
Change Is the Law of Life

"If we want things to stay as they are, things will have to change."

—Giuseppe di Lampedusa in his poetic study of French society, The Leopard.

Change is as much a part of life as breathing. If only it was as simple, too! The truth is, change is hard at first. Like playing the piano, change requires daily practice. You make mistakes, maybe a lot at first, but you get better and better. Before you know it, that run of sixteenth notes that once tripped your fingers now flows without effort.

You're probably not too concerned about French society, and maybe not even about playing the piano. But we know you're concerned about changing your life for the health of your heart. So let's get started. Before you know it, you'll be making heart-healthy choices without a second thought.

Chapter 20

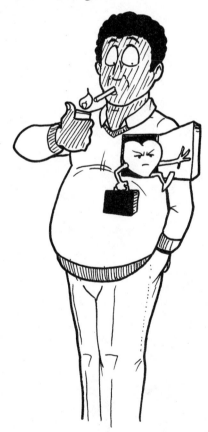

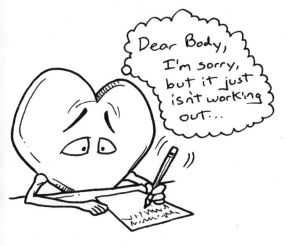

The Heart Has Its Reasons

In This Chapter

➤ Identifying your life's risk level: A self-quiz

➤ Why you make the choices you do

➤ Planning for successful (permanent) change

"It is only by risking our persons from one hour to another that we live at all," wrote American philosopher William James. Indeed, living is a process of choosing risks. A funny thing about risk is that often what we perceive as the most dangerous is the least likely to happen. And what we neglect can have the most serious consequence. What do you fear most, being in a plane crash or a car crash? Most of us fear a plane crash far more yet are thousands of times more likely to be involved in a car crash—and more than a third of us fail to buckle up when we get in the car. Some risks are such steady habits that you might not even recognize them for the dangers they present.

Are You a Risk-Taker?: A Lifestyle Self-Quiz

How close to the edge do you live? Take this little quiz to find out! Pick the answer that best describes what *you* would do:

1. I wear a seat belt in my car...

    A. Always.

    B. When I drive.

    C. If I'm going farther than five miles.

    D. Only when I see a cop.

2. I cross against the signal...

    A. Hardly ever.

    B. When I'm in a hurry and I can see there are no cars coming.

    C. When it takes too long to change; as long as I'm in the crosswalk, I have the right of way.

    D. What signal?

Cardio Care

It's tempting—and human nature, say researchers who study human behavior—to test your risk limits. People who take cholesterol-lowering drugs, for example, might feel "safe" continuing unhealthy eating habits because they believe the medication protects them from high blood cholesterol. This is false security. Reducing your risk through medication is certainly easier (and more expensive), but lifestyle still gives you the best overall chance at good health.

3. I drive the speed limit...

    A. Almost always.

    B. In town and in school zones.

    C. When there's a police car behind me.

    D. As long as I'm not in a hurry.

4. The stoplight just turned yellow. That's my signal to...

    A. Start slowing down.

    B. Turn down a side street to take another route.

    C. Creep closer and closer to the intersection so I can shoot through as soon as the light turns green.

    D. Floor it—I don't have time to sit around waiting for a red light.

5. The sun's out and I've got nothing to do today but enjoy it. I put on sunscreen...

    A. Before I go out and every couple hours.

    B. On places where a sunburn would hurt.

    C. After I've been out for a while and notice my skin feels hot.

    D. Don't use the stuff; been out in the sun all my life without it, why change now?

Tally the As, Bs, Cs, and Ds that you circled. If four or more of your answers are As and Bs, you do a pretty good job of managing your everyday risks. Three or more Cs, and you're walking the edge. Two or more Ds, and you're flirting with a shortened lifespan. Look a little closer at your own life. What are your three most risky behaviors?

My three most risky behaviors are

1. _____

2. _____

3. _____

Yeah, but what's this got to do with my heart, you ask? Odds are, plenty. The more risks you take in general, the more risks you're likely to be taking with your heart health, too. Risk can be a (dangerous) lifestyle. So let's narrow our focus and take a quick look at the risks you take with your heart health:

1. My weight has crept up a few pounds over the years. It's time to...

   A. Start walking at lunchtime.

   B. Trade some of those steaks for chicken and fish.

   C. Pass on a third helping of those mashed potatoes and gravy, even though they're really good.

   D. Go shopping for clothes that fit.

2. I'm going to a wedding this weekend, and I know there's going to be a buffet brunch at the reception. I'd do well to...

   A. Eat a turkey sandwich before I leave, so I'm not famished by the time the buffet starts.

   B. Start with salads and bread, then go back for an entrée.

   C. Take some of everything I think I might want, just in case they run out before I get back to the buffet line.

   D. Eat as much as I can hold, since brunch covers two meals (and besides, some one else is footing the bill).

3. My father and his two sisters have high blood pressure. Since I know this runs in families, I'm...

   A. Keeping my weight down and my activity level up.

   B. Using breathing techniques and yoga to manage my stress.

   C. Checking my blood pressure at one of those machines every time I go to the drugstore.

   D. Not worried. If it's in my genes, what can I do?

4. I went to a health fair, and they told me my cholesterol is 320. I should...

   A. Schedule an appointment with my doctor to find out what this means.

   B. Start walking at lunchtime.

   C. Give up chocolate and potato chips.

   D. Ignore it. Those "quickie" tests don't tell you anything.

5. I suddenly feel lightheaded, and my hands and legs feel heavy. Just when I'm starting to worry, it stops. I...

   A. Recognize this could be an early warning sign of stroke or ministroke and call my doctor or hospital emergency room for advice.

   B. Sit down right away, so I don't fall and hurt myself.

   C. Think about calling the doctor, but decide to wait to see if it happens again.

   D. Go on with whatever I was doing. What's a little lightheadedness?

Red Alert!
Remember, early treatment is the key to surviving a stroke or heart attack. Seek prompt medical attention if you have signs of either. Treatment (especially clot-busters) is most effective in the first hours of a heart attack or stroke. Delay can increase the severity of damage or cost you your life.

How did you do on these risks? Again, if you're mostly in the As and Bs, you know your heart health risks and are taking steps to reduce them. Three or more Cs? Your heart's in the right place, but your actions aren't helping it stay there. Two or more Ds, and you're courting a coronary. Again, take a close look at your personal life. What three behaviors put *your* heart at risk?

My personal three heart-risking behaviors are

1. _____

2. _____

3. _____

Why You Do the Things You Do

Even people who know better make unhealthy choices. Another $64,000 question! To some extent, it's just human nature. Each time you take a risk and fail to suffer the threatened consequence, you're emboldened to take that risk again. And again. Nothing's going to happen—you're living proof. The longer you defy a particular risk, the easier it is to believe you can always do so.

Can you remember the first time you crossed in the middle of a busy street? Your heart was pounding and your mouth dry by the time you reached the other side, even though the closest car in sight was at least a block away. What about now? Most likely, you don't even run, knowing that drivers who honk their horns at least see you and aren't very likely to run you down. What does it take to make you change your ways? Often, only immediate danger. The first time a car nearly clips you because the driver was looking for a radio station will likely end your jaywalking, at least till the memories that flashed before your eyes settle back into their places.

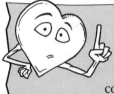

Take It to Heart

We fear cancer more than we fear heart disease, even though heart disease kills more Americans each year than do all forms of cancer combined.

Looking Beyond Here and Now

It's 10pm and there's no milk for tomorrow's breakfast. No problem—the local food mart's open around the clock for your shopping convenience. You've worked hard all day, and you're starving. No problem—there are at least a half dozen fast-food options between work and home. In the mood for a new car? No problem—sign a few papers, and the keys are yours.

When we can have what we want *now*, it's hard to see any farther. And it's natural to go for what makes you feel good today, right now. After all, who knows what tomorrow will bring? Sure, you know a diet high in fat threatens your heart. But you ate a double side of bacon yesterday, and you're still among the living. One adventure with a double side of bacon may have no immediate consequences beyond indigestion. It's especially easy to be careless with risks when the consequences are distant and cumulative. When it comes to making changes, we want to see immediate results.

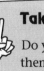

Take It to Heart

Do you make New Year's resolutions every year, only to abandon them before the year's first month is over? Give yourself a little more time. While some changes might come easily, it can take a couple months or even a couple years to transition from a familiar to a new behavior. Break major changes into smaller, manageable goals—"walk for 20 minutes at lunch time," for example, rather than "work out at the gym for two hours after work." Gradual change over time is more effective—and more likely to be permanent.

The Best Intentions

It's not that we mean to make unhealthy choices. It's just that there's such a gap between what we intend and what we do. We try, really we do. Eight million Americans participate in weight-loss programs. We spend billions of dollars on home-exercise equipment and fitness-club memberships. Yet a third of us are overweight and out of shape. And a million of us will die as a direct result of our unhealthy habits.

The problem is, we're still looking for that fast fix and it doesn't exist. Change is a process of growth that takes time. Change doesn't happen all at once. It happens in stages. Sure, at some point, it'll seem like you lost 20 pounds overnight. But you really didn't. You dropped a pound or so a week for nearly five months. Which was what you intended to do, wasn't it?

Information Overload

Sometimes it's just overwhelming to think about all the things you should do to live a healthy life. The things you already do, you don't think about—you just do them. We live in a time when the last thing we need more of is information. Remember the exercise of trying to chew a French fry 20 or 30 times? Extracting substance from the "sound bites" that bombard us day in and day out is just about as futile. So we stick with what we know; it's less confusing.

Was Darwin Right About Evolution?

By Heart

Evolution is the process by which plants and animals change in response to changes in their environments. *Natural selection* describes the way stronger or more adaptable individuals within a species survive and pass their genes to future generations. Weaker individuals are unable to survive and don't reproduce, eliminating their genes from future generations. Both terms apply to genes, not individuals.

Though it was Charles Darwin who upended the biological theory of his time when he published *On the Origin of Species* in 1859, other scientists had made similar observations. In a process known as *evolution,* animal and plant species change in response to environmental changes. Darwin further theorized that the species that survive through such changes are genetically stronger than those that don't. (Doesn't it seem that those dandelions come back stronger and in greater numbers every spring?) What Darwin and scientists call *natural selection,* the rest of us know as *survival of the fittest.* In a modern context, scientists include the behavioral choices an individual makes among the factors that influence the selection process.

Do Only the Strong Survive?

Consider the most rapidly growing segment of our population, people over age 85. While your chance of dying increases significantly for each year after age 50, the rate at which it does so decreases after age 85 or so. People who live into their 90s and beyond often suffer from hearing loss and cataracts. But contrary to popular perception, few have debilitating medical conditions. When those over 85 end up in nursing homes, it's generally because of a single precipitating event, like a heart attack or a broken hip. Could it be that only the strong survive? Scientists believe that genes and heartiness play definite roles in longevity. In fact, genetics appears to play a much larger role in many health outcomes than scientists imagined. Genes appear to influence your levels of HDL and LDL cholesterol, for example, and your levels of *homocysteine* (a cell waste product that affects your cholesterol). Both are risk factors for heart disease. Such discoveries give scientists hope that in the future, gene therapy can end hereditary risk factors for many diseases.

Take It to Heart

Gene therapy—altering the genetic structure of diseased cells—holds great promise for treating and even curing many debilitating conditions, like muscular dystrophy and cystic fibrosis. Researchers are also studying the role genetic engineering might play in treating acquired conditions like cancer, diabetes, and even heart disease. Don't rush to your doctor for a gene transplant, though. Real-world use of these high-tech techniques is more likely to be an option for your children and grandchildren than for you.

Finding the Courage to Change

It's not easy to change. Old habits feel good, no matter how bad they can be for you. Change feels funny. It's new, different, and uncertain. How do you know that what you're moving to is better than what you're leaving behind? Even when the evidence seems irrefutable, you still have doubts. Will it work for me? Will my efforts make a difference? Can I really go through with it? The answer can be "yes" to all these questions. A good place to start is with the list of your three heart-risking behaviors that you just wrote down. Select one that you think you could change. Here are some tips to help you build a solid bridge between your intentions and your actions:

➤ **Take one step at a time.** This is your life, not your living room. You can't change your habits like you change your décor.

➤ **Change is give and take.** Don't just give something up. It won't last. Replace the unhealthy habit with a healthy one. Whatever you do now, you're doing it because you need to.

Just for YOU

Do you have risks for heart disease that you cannot change, such as family history or diabetes? Then it's all the more important for you to manage the risks you *can* change. While such "risk management" is a lifelong process, it's never too late to start.

➤ **Write down your goals and an action plan for reaching them.** This helps you think through what you want to change and how you're going to do it.

➤ **Draw support from friends and family.** Once you've decided to make a change, tell your loved ones. Maybe they'll join you in your new habit. At the very least, they can offer support and encouragement.

➤ **Reward yourself.** Give yourself a special treat when you reach a goal. Go to a concert, take in a movie, buy a book.

Living to Your Heart's Content

Living a heart-healthy lifestyle doesn't mean you have to give up everything you enjoy in life. What would be the point? On the other hand, it doesn't make much sense to set yourself up for early death from heart disease, either. Sure, you've spent a lifetime indulging in the heart-hurting risks that are now your lifestyle. But you have the rest of your life to adopt heart-healthy changes. And you might find that doing so gains you far more than you give up.

How much of your present lifestyle is actually the result of choices you've made after weighing the consequences of all the options available to you? Odds are, very little. Choosing a heart-healthy lifestyle gives you the chance to take control of your life, to make choices that keep your heart in mind. And who knows? You might actually enjoy your choices!

The Least You Need to Know

➤ Even with "good" genes, you have to make healthy choices.

➤ Though it may seem like it takes a long time to see the results of your changes, your heart feels them right away.

➤ Successful change takes planning and practice. It doesn't happen overnight.

➤ While modern medicine can help, lifestyle changes can make the difference between heart trouble and heart health.

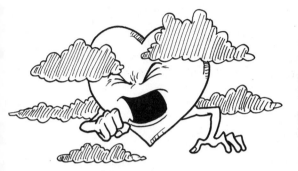

Light Up Your Heart, Not a Cigarette

In This Chapter

➤ The addictive power of cigarette smoking

➤ The health costs of smoking

➤ The danger of secondhand smoke

➤ How to quit smoking for good

Americans spend $50 billion on tobacco products a year; $47 billion on cigarettes alone. The United States government subsidizes crop insurance for tobacco farmers to the tune of $40 million a year. Yet tobacco products have no known health benefits and dozens of unhealthy consequences. So why does a quarter of our country's population light up every day?

Smoking: Why the Whole World Is Hooked

The reason people keep smoking is not the same reason they start. Most people start smoking for a variety of reasons—to look and feel "cool" or more grown up, because "everyone" else does, to control weight, because they like the taste or smell of cigarette smoke. But they keep smoking because cigarettes contain a physically *addictive* drug called *nicotine*.

By Heart

Addiction occurs when your body becomes dependent upon a substance. *Nicotine* is an addictive drug present in tobacco. A stimulant, nicotine causes your brain to release higher levels of *dopamine*, a chemical substance that causes feelings of pleasure. When you are physically addicted, your body experiences unpleasant symptoms when you stop taking the substance.

Nicotine reaches your brain within a minute of entering your bloodstream, where it stimulates nerve activity. This often causes a feeling of alertness. It also increases the levels of *dopamine* in your brain, a chemical related to feelings of pleasure. This part of your brain's not particularly smart, and it likes these feelings. When it doesn't get them, it sends annoying signals that your body interprets as "Light a cigarette, now!"

While people react in varying ways to the effects of nicotine, nearly every smoker who quits goes through some degree of withdrawal. Sometimes this is little more than drowsiness and headaches. Sometimes it includes agitation, irritability, and other, more unpleasant, effects. Physically, it takes your body about two weeks to completely rid itself of nicotine. This is longer than many smokers can hold out. One in ten of the 20 million Americans who stop smoking this year will be smoke-free next year.

Take It to Heart

Smoking's been around practically since the discovery of fire. Until the 1880s, anyone who wanted to light up had to roll his (or her) own. Then cigarette-making joined the age of industrialization and became a symbol of status. Heroes from the front lines of two world wars to the box office lineups of Hollywood flashed smiles and cigarettes. Popularity peaked in the 1960s, when television introduced a new generation to smoking. The federal Public Health Cigarette Smoking Act of 1969 put an end to cigarette ads on TV and radio, and the number of smokers started dropping.

The Numbers Tell the Story

Since the U.S. Surgeon General first issued a public health warning about the dangers of smoking in 1964, tobacco use has become the leading preventable cause of death in the United States. It has claimed the lives of more than 10 million Americans. Did you "come of age" and start smoking around the time this first warning hit the papers? If you've smoked the average of one pack a day since then, you've coated your lungs with about seven pounds of tar (some of which they've been able to hack out, thanks to your smoker's cough). If you laid the equivalent number of unsmoked cigarettes end to end, they'd cover about 11 miles. Statistics show:

➤ 48 million Americans over the age of 18 smoke.

➤ 4.4 million young people, ages 12 to 17, smoke. Each day, 3,000 more join them.

➤ Smoking kills nearly 1,200 people each day, one in five of them from heart disease.

➤ If you smoke, you can expect to die seven years earlier than if you didn't.

➤ Tobacco use accounts for more than $50 billion in medical costs each year. We all pay for these costs, smokers and nonsmokers alike, through higher health insurance premiums.

What Do You Know About Smoking?: A Self-Quiz

The statistics show the big picture of smoking. But what do you know about how smoking affects you? Answer these questions to find out!

		True	False
1.	I could vacation for a week in Hawaii for what it costs to support a pack-a-day smoking habit for a year.	_____	_____
2.	I've smoked all my life, so there's no point in quitting now.	_____	_____
3.	I'm young. Smoking won't be a problem for me for years, and I'll quit by then so it won't matter.	_____	_____
4.	I smoke cigars, so I don't inhale. This protects me from smoking's harmful effects.	_____	_____
5.	I don't care about all the doom and gloom. I like smoking, and I'm going to continue. What I do, whether it's bad for me or not, is my business.	_____	_____

If you answered True to number 1 and False to everything else, congratulations! Here's the lowdown:

1. **True.** The average pack of cigarettes sells for $2.25. At a pack a day, you're sending more than $800 a year up in smoke. Depending on where you live, that could be more than enough for a few days in the sun.

2. **False.** No matter how long you've smoked, there are health benefits from quitting. Obviously, if you wait until you have heart disease, lung disease, or cancer, you're not going to be like new a year after you throw away the cigarettes. But if you stop *before* these conditions develop, after a year, your risk of heart disease drops by half and in about 10 years, to that of someone who never smoked.

3. **False.** Quitting is your best option, no matter what your age. The longer you smoke, the more damage you do to your body and the more likely it is that at least some of

219

it will be permanent. While the benefits of not smoking start 20 minutes after your last puff, the longer you smoke, the more likely you are to develop smoking-related health problems that are not so easy to reverse.

Cardio Care
Like to see evidence of your progress as you move toward becoming a nonsmoker? Get a glass jar and put it on your counter. Each time you would've bought a pack of cigarettes, put the money in the jar instead. You'll see your "smoke stash" grow, showing you what you're saving (besides your health) by giving up cigarettes.

4. **False.** Your tissues absorb nicotine and other chemicals from the smoke swirling in your mouth. One fat stogie that you nurse along for an hour or so packs as much nicotine as an entire pack of cigarettes. (Smokeless tobacco products also deliver nicotine.) People who smoke cigars regularly also have a higher risk of mouth and throat cancer.

5. **False.** Hummm. Well, yes, you should be able to make choices, good or bad, about how to live your life. The problem is, your decision to smoke affects others—the people around you who breathe in what you blow out, and everyone who pays social security or health insurance premiums. Three thousand people a year die from lung cancer caused by substances unique to cigarette smoke, even though they've never lit up. And as a country, we spend more than $50 billion for medical care for health problems that smoking causes.

Every Puff You Take: What Smoking Does

Every puff from a cigarette carries more than 4,000 chemicals into your lungs, at least 43 of which cause cancer. Some are so poisonous that possessing them requires a special permit, like DDT (an insecticide) and arsenic. These substances affect every cell in your body in some way, from your skin to your heart.

To Your Heart

Two things happen to your heart right away when you light up a cigarette:

➤ Carbon monoxide replaces oxygen in the red blood cells that leave your lungs, shortchanging your heart of the vital energy source that fuels its work.

➤ Nicotine stimulates your brain, leading it to signal your heart to pick up the pace. So your heart beats faster and harder, even though your body's demands for oxygen and nutrients haven't increased.

And from the minute nicotine enters your bloodstream, it affects your blood vessels, causing them to stiffen and become less flexible. This becomes a big deal when the vessels are your *coronary arteries* (supplying blood to your heart) and your *aorta* (the conduit carrying blood from your heart to the rest of your body). Your heart has to work harder to send blood through stiff, inflexible arteries, which raises your blood pressure. It takes about 20 minutes for these effects to wear off. Their temporary nature doesn't save you from long-term damage, though.

Repeated exposure to nicotine eventually wears your arteries down, and they develop microscopic ruptures or rips in their walls. Though the leaks that result are so tiny you don't notice any blood loss, your body does. It sends *platelets* (clotting cells) rushing to the rescue, where they pile on to plug the damage. They stay in the form of clots until the wounds heal. During this time, the clots act like magnets for fatty deposits, which glob on. These deposits stay even after the clots disappear, increasing your risk for heart attack or stroke.

To Your Lungs

Whoa, do your lungs cringe when they see that smoke rolling their way! Your millions of alveoli would close up and hide if they could. But they can't, so instead, they fill with tar and other residues that smoke leaves behind. No problem, though—you have that lovely smoker's hack to try to clear it away. Well, actually it *is* a problem, over time. Those residues bury the little *cilia* (the hair-like brushes that sweep gunk out of your lungs and up to your bronchia so you can cough it out). The alveoli eventually rupture, further diminishing their ability to exchange oxygen for carbon dioxide and other wastes.

The continual irritation of all this rubs your lungs raw inside, so they form scar tissue to try to heal themselves. This irritation also sets the stage for cancer to develop. And all those other substances that smoke contains crowd oxygen aside, giving your lungs less than they need. So every cell in your body gets shortchanged, because your blood can't deliver what it doesn't have.

> **Red Alert!**
> So you've tried to quit but slipped? Don't panic. The typical smoker makes three to five attempts before becoming a nonsmoker for good. Just be patient with yourself. Try to identify what triggered your momentary lapse, give yourself three ways to resist the temptation if it arises again, and move on. Every time you try to quit, you get closer to success!

To Your Whole Body

Remember the childhood song "the anklebone's connected to the leg bone, the leg bone's connected to the…"? When it comes to smoking, what enters your lungs is connected to every part of your body in some way. In addition to your heart and lungs, smoking leaves no part of your body untouched:

➤ **Brain:** Nicotine is a stimulant that increases your brain's activity. After a while, your brain depends on this stimulation and sends signals in the form of cravings when it doesn't get enough.

➤ **Muscles:** Your muscles need oxygen to work well. Smoking shortchanges them by sending carbon monoxide instead, and they tire faster. Your muscles also release lactic acid and other byproducts of metabolism more slowly, since the red blood cells that carry these waste materials away can't take them on.

➤ **Skin:** The chemicals in cigarette smoke destroy your skin's *elastin*, a stretchy substance that keeps wrinkles at bay. Because smoking damages your *capillaries*, the thread-like blood vessels that deliver oxygen and nutrients to your body tissues, smoking prevents nourishment from reaching your skin cells.

Red Alert!
Don't think you're off the hook if smokeless tobacco or chewing is your habit. No matter what its form, tobacco releases nicotine (and cancer-causing substances) into your body. Whether it comes from smoking or chewing, over time, nicotine damages your arteries.

➤ **Mouth:** The worst thing about bad breath is that you're usually the last person to know you have it. But bad breath's the least of your mouth worries as a smoker. Tar from cigarette smoke stains your teeth. Nicotine and other chemicals in smoke irritate your gums, tongue, and cheek tissues, causing dental problems and possibly mouth and throat cancer.

➤ **Digestive system:** The constant invasion of chemicals and cancer-causing substances that smoking subjects your body to raises your risk of ordinarily rare cancers of the liver, stomach, and pancreas. Smoking also dulls your taste buds and your sense of smell.

Take It to Heart

Worried about gaining weight if you quit smoking? Don't! The average weight gain for smokers who make no other changes is about 5 pounds, mostly because they munch instead. If you add half an hour of physical activity to your daily routine, like a walk at lunchtime, you'll more than offset this small amount.

Secondhand Smoke Is No Joke

Tobacco companies will remember the 1990s as the decade of secondhand smoke. In 1993, the *Environmental Protection Agency* (EPA) designated secondhand smoke, also called *environmental tobacco smoke,* as a *group A carcinogen* (a substance directly capable of causing cancer). Nonsmokers with smoking-related cancers filed dozens of lawsuits charging tobacco companies with accountability for their illnesses. Some won, resulting in the first major changes in more than 20 years in the ways companies market and sell tobacco products.

For You and the Ones You Love

Despite the growing number of smoke-free environments, nine of ten Americans still face regular exposure to secondhand smoke. You might work in an office or building where employers permit smoking, or wait for a bus surrounded by others puffing away to get in a smoke before the bus pulls up. Do you smoke? Where? How many other people "smoke" because you do? Many smokers only smoke outside, even in their own homes. This protects others from secondhand smoke and often reduces the number of cigarettes you smoke (especially when it's cold and wet outside).

Kids' Hearts and Health at Risk

Many of those who deal with secondhand smoke are children who live with smoking parents. These children have more ear infections and upper respiratory infections than children who live in smoke-free homes. Secondhand smoke sends 20 infants to the hospital every day for more serious lower respiratory infections like pneumonia. And every hour, secondhand smoke triggers asthma attacks in 23 children. There's mounting evidence that regular exposure to secondhand smoke affects your arteries the same as if you had smoked those cigarettes yourself. We don't know about you, but we find the mental image of a three-year-old puffing away on a cigarette appalling. If you smoke, quit. If you're not going to quit, at least don't force your kids to smoke, too. They'll thank you from the bottom of their hearts.

Just for YOU

If you're pregnant and you smoke, your baby smokes, too. The chemicals in tobacco smoke enter your baby's bloodstream nearly as quickly as they enter yours, and can have serious health consequences. Smoking reduces the amount of oxygen that reaches your baby's developing organs. At birth, the babies of smoking moms are often underweight (which can cause a variety of health problems for the baby), and have narrowed airways and reduced lung function.

Cardio Care

Children who live with adults who smoke are significantly more likely to have upper respiratory infections, asthma, and ear infections than children who live in smoke-free homes.

How You Can Quit Smoking for Good

Got a lot of experience quitting? Most smokers do. The typical smoker stops smoking at least once a year, at least for a day. The best way to quit smoking, of course, is never to start. An estimated 42 million Americans who once considered smoking decided not to as a result of antismoking education. Of the 48 million who made the other choice, nearly half will give up their habit for at least a day. Sadly, 90 percent will return to it within a year.

So how do you count yourself among the lucky two million who succeed? Start by surrounding yourself with nonsmoking family and friends who can support you. Remove

> **Cardio Care**
> To get a handle on when you smoke, keep a daily log for a few days. Then try to cut the number of cigarettes you smoke in half. Stay at that level for two weeks (the amount of time it takes your body to adjust to the new nicotine dose). Repeat this cycle until you're smoking so few cigarettes in a day, it's hardly worth the effort.

all accouterments of smoking from your home, car, purse, workshop, office, boat, motor home—anywhere you stash "one, just in case." Get rid of cigarettes, ashtrays, lighters, and even matches. If you usually eat or drink before, during, or after smoking, try to get the items you're most likely to associate with smoking out of your life, too. (Though don't throw out your spouse if you usually light up after sex— there are other, less drastic, measures you can substitute!) The idea is to remove temptation—while out of sight won't necessarily be out of mind, it is out of reach.

Forget about any ceremonial last smoke—you're celebrating the start of a new lifestyle, not mourning the end of a former one. Celebrate the first time you would've had a cigarette and didn't! Attitude is critical. If you want to join the 10 percent who stay smoke-free, you have to see life without cigarettes as more desirable than life with them.

> **Take It to Heart**
> The more you prepare for your transition from a smoking to a nonsmoking lifestyle, the more likely you are to succeed. If you've tried to quit a number of times before, consider making *this* effort your strongest ever. Have your carpets, drapes, and even furniture cleaned to remove all traces of cigarette smoke from your home. If it's been a while since you've redecorated, this is the perfect opportunity to repaint, too. The desire to keep your "new" home clean might be the added incentive you need to stay smoke-free.

Nicotine-Replacement Therapy

> **Cardio Care**
> What's the *first* thing you do when you get up in the morning? Do you light a cigarette? If so, your addiction to nicotine is high. You'll find nicotine-replacement gum or patches a big help in your efforts to quit smoking.

Nicotine-replacement therapy substitutes another source of nicotine for the source you've thrown away. These products, commonly available as gum, skin patches, and nasal spray, ease your body's withdrawal from nicotine by giving it just enough to take the edge off. This helps you make it through the first weeks with less discomfort. People who use nicotine-replacement therapy in the early stages of smoking cessation are twice as likely to continue their efforts to quit than those people who don't use the therapy. You can buy many of these products without a prescription. Of course, at some point, you have to stop these products, too. Because they deliver nicotine more slowly and consistently, your brain doesn't get quite the rush from them that it does from cigarettes. This makes it easier to gradually taper off nicotine replacements.

"Do I Need a Program to Succeed?"

Not necessarily, though smoking-cessation programs are often helpful. The American Heart Association, American Lung Association, American Cancer Society, and most hospitals can direct you to effective programs in your area. Smoking-cessation programs help you identify the reasons you smoke and find ways to address them. They also provide a good support group of people going through the same experiences you are.

Other Quitting Aids

Smokers who want to quit are often willing to try anything that sounds like it can help. Again, we come back to the old caution: Like any other "quick-fix" solutions, if it sounds too good to be true, it probably is. And the more it costs, the more likely it is too good to be true! In reality, despite the benefits, quitting is a challenge. If the clerk hands you a pack of your regular brand along with your change at the gas station, you've been smoking long enough for your body to resist your efforts to stop. Aids that are most helpful are those that can become a regular, long-term part of your new lifestyle—breathing techniques, exercise, and meditation are all ways to replace smoking with more healthful activities.

Getting the Upper Hand on Those Pesky Cravings

You've quit smoking, but you can't shake that desperate desire to light up a cigarette. Though it might seem like it lasts an eternity, your craving will disappear in about two minutes—whether you smoke or not. Make a list of 10 things you can do instead of smoking, and carry it with you. Do something from your list—pet the cat, go for a walk around the block, whatever will take your mind off smoking. When the craving passes, pat yourself on the back. You've made it past another trigger!

Your Personal Stop-Smoking Plan

If all it took to give up smoking was understanding how smoking destroys your health, you'd all be non-smokers by now. But it's not that easy, as those of you who smoke know all too well.

If you smoke, take a few minutes right now to sketch out a plan to stop smoking.

Cardio Care
If you haven't been able to quit despite lots of good determination and advice, you've tried everything you can think of, and even nicotine replacement doesn't seem to help, you could be dealing with anxiety or depression. Everyone smokes because it makes them feel good and makes stress less noticeable-for a few minutes. But if you haven't been able to quit and think you might be anxious or depressed, talk to your doctor about other quitting aids, in particular anti-depressant medications like doxepin or bupropion (Zyban®) that help some smokers quit.

225

I want to stop smoking because:

1. _____

2. _____

3. _____

4. _____

5. _____

I'm most tempted to smoke when:

1. _____

2. _____

3. _____

4. _____

5. _____

Instead of smoking, I can:

1. _____

2. _____

3. _____

4. _____

5. _____

My quit date is: _____

With the money I save by not buying cigarettes, I want to: _____

_____

The Least You Need to Know

➤ Smoking is an addiction (both physical and psychological) that requires support and determination to stop.

➤ Smoking affects every cell in your body in some way.

➤ It's never too late to quit smoking. Your body begins to benefit 20 minutes after your last cigarette.

➤ Secondhand smoke is a serious health problem, especially for children who live in homes with adults who smoke.

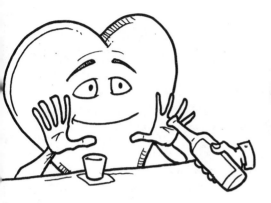

An Unnatural High

Our society is very drug oriented. Medications offer a fix for almost anything that ails us. Our favorite foods and drinks contain mind- and sometimes body-altering substances. Sometimes you don't even know that what you've ingested is, or contains, a drug. But your heart does.

Does a Drink a Day Keep Heart Attacks Away?

The short answer: We don't know for sure. A number of studies suggest that moderate alcohol consumption helps protect against heart disease by raising HDL (good) cholesterol and reducing plaque accumulations in your arteries. Alcohol also has a mild anti-coagulating effect, keeping platelets from clumping together to form clots in your arteries. Both processes reduce the risk of heart attack. How strongly alcohol influences either, and in what ways, remains uncertain.

Take It to Heart

Interest in alcohol as a treatment for heart disease is nothing new.

"Of all remedies in threatening death by cardiac failure, Spirits are the best, being at once available, convenient, rapid in their action, and almost invariably successful if recovery be possible. Hardly less valuable is Alcohol, given continuously in small regular doses, in chronic disease of the heart... Wine, Rectified Spirit, or various Tinctures may be prescribed in such cases."

So advised physician and medical professor J. Mitchell Bruce in his 1884 handbook, *Materia Medica and Therapeutics, an Introduction to the Rational Treatment of Disease.* Alcohol also found favor as a treatment for sleeplessness, dental pain, water retention, and fever reduction.

"The French Paradox"

French cardiologist Dr. Serge Renaud conducted the largest study about the role of alcohol and heart disease in an attempt to explain "the French paradox"—how French citizens could eat diets brimming with saturated fats yet have very little heart disease. His extensive study of 34,000 middle-aged men concluded that the wine the men drank with their meals offset the potential damage of the meat, cheese, and butter central to their diets. Dr. Renaud reported his findings in 1991, setting off an enormous controversy.

Take It to Heart

Matters of the heart aside, what's moderate for one person could be legally intoxicating for someone else. Responding to concerns about drunk driving, many states now consider a person to be intoxicated with a blood-alcohol level of 0.08 percent. If you're physically small, say 5'3" and 107 pounds, two glasses of wine with dinner could put you over the legal limit.

What Is Moderate?

The key factor is *moderate*, a concept that's difficult to pin down to an amount. Dr. Renaud's study participants drank two or three glasses of wine a day, the equivalent of 20 to 30 grams of alcohol. One drink a day, every day, is very different than seven drinks just on one day, even though both average out to a drink a day for the week. (For one thing, seven drinks in a short time could contain enough alcohol to poison you.)

Whether you're a man or a woman makes a difference, too. By nature's design, a woman's body contains more fat and less water than a man's. Water draws alcohol, so those few beers leave a man's body faster than they leave a woman's. Both men and women gain body fat with aging, too, so the older you are, the less efficiently your body metabolizes alcohol.

How Alcohol Affects Your Heart

Despite the apparent benefits of moderate alcohol consumption, heavy alcohol use, particularly over time, can damage your heart. Half the people who drink heavily (more than three drinks a day) have high blood pressure, which can lead to coronary disease, congestive heart failure, and stroke. The older you are, the more likely you'll be among them (though these risks are somewhat reversible if you stop drinking).

Heavy drinking also causes a direct decrease in heart muscle strength. Since alcohol's calories are empty, your body converts them to fat almost immediately. Heavy drinking puts more fat into circulation in your body, raising your triglyceride level.

A serious alcohol-related heart problem is alcoholic *cardiomyopathy* (enlarged heart). Because long-term heavy drinking also damages other organs, like your liver and brain, people with alcoholic cardiomyopathy often don't respond well to the medications generally used to treat this condition. And because of other organ damage, they're not good candidates for the treatment of last resort, a heart transplant.

Weighing the Risks and the Benefits

Several dozen studies conducted or reported since Dr. Renaud startled the medical community with his prescription for daily wine have confirmed that light to moderate drinking can benefit your heart. So why do doctors hesitate to recommend a drink a day to prevent heart disease if there's all that evidence? The line separating healthful from unhealthy is hard to walk— and sometimes even hard to find. Alcohol abuse exacts

Cardio Care
The departments of Agriculture and Health and Human Services define *moderate drinking* as no more than one drink a day for women and two drinks a day for men. A drink, according to the guidelines, is roughly 12 grams ($1/2$ ounce) of absolute alcohol. A 5-ounce glass of wine, 12-ounce bottle of beer, and $1/2$ ounce distilled spirits (80 proof) all contain about this amount of alcohol.

Red Alert!
Heavy drinking (more than three drinks a day on a regular basis) affects your body's ability to stop bleeding. A liver damaged by alcohol has trouble making clotting proteins. Also, your body can't keep enough platelets, which it also needs to stop bleeding, in circulation. Further compounding the problem, an unhealthy liver creates abnormal pressure on some veins near your stomach and esophagus, making them likely to burst and cause a life-threatening bleeding episode.

a terrible toll from its victims, their families, and our communities. Drunk drivers kill more than 17,000 Americans each year and injure a million more. Medical conditions resulting from alcohol abuse—cirrhosis and other liver diseases, psychiatric problems, nutritional deficiencies, injuries from accidents, and alcohol poisoning—drain more than $45 billion a year from our healthcare system. (That's the equivalent of $1 for every drink consumed.) Health care providers would rather see you eat right, exercise regularly, and maintain a healthy weight to control your risks for heart disease.

By Heart

Cardio-myopathy is a potentially serious disorder in which the heart muscle weakens and the heart becomes enlarged. Some forms of this disease, such as alcoholic cardiomyopathy, have a clear cause. Rarely, cardiomyopathy occurs for no apparent reason. This is called "idiopathic," which means "of unknown cause." The larger the heart becomes, the less effectively it pumps.

Cardio Care

The American Heart Association recommends caution in using alcohol to lower your risk for heart disease until we know more about alcohol's effects on the heart. If you drink now, do so moderately—no more than one or two drinks a day. If you don't drink now, don't start just for your heart.

How Much Do You Drink, and Why?: A Self-Quiz

How much do you drink now? Sometimes it's hard to see whether your drinking level is light, moderate, or heavy until it's in front of you in black and white. Try this quiz to measure your level:

1. It's Friday night, and a bunch of us are going out after work. I'll probably drink…

   A. A beer or glass of wine with dinner.

   B. A pitcher of beer while we shoot some pool or throw darts.

   C. Tequila shooters.

   D. Until I puke or pass out, whichever comes first.

2. It's Saturday morning. I feel…

   A. Great! The sun's out, the birds are singing, and I'm happy to be alive!

   B. Like I'll sleep in for a while.

   C. How much coffee does it take to sober up?

   D. Like a drink. Put a shot of vodka in that orange juice, wouldja?

3. It's my birthday. To celebrate, I think I'll…

   A. Go out to dinner with family and friends, maybe have a glass of expensive wine or champagne.

   B. Pick up a case of beer and have some friends over.

   C. Buy a round for all my buddies and anyone else who happens to be at the Drink-'Til-You-Drop Lounge.

D. Stay home and put a serious dent in that bottle of scotch I've been saving for a special occasion.

4. The folks (or the kids) are coming for a weekend visit. Before they get here, I need to...

    A. Put clean sheets on the bed in the guest room.

    B. Go grocery shopping so there's actually food in the fridge.

    C. Take all those wine bottles and beer cans to the recycle center.

    D. Stash a few bottles of brandy in my bedroom, in case I want a nightcap.

5. My best friend got married last night. The reception was a blast, because...

    A. I had a great time catching up with friends and family I haven't seen for a while.

    B. The no-host bar was free.

    C. Everyone was soused, so no one noticed when I fell down the steps trying to throw rice.

    D. I went to a wedding last night? Please tell me it wasn't mine!

6. Man, what a day. A flat tire, the computer crashed, the fire drill was real, I just know that blueberry's gonna stain, and the cat turned my new drapes into blinds. Time to unwind with...

    A. An extra hour in the gym to sweat out all that stress, then some meditation before bed.

    B. Bowling and a couple beers.

    C. A bottle of wine and the rest of that chocolate cake.

    D. A good slug right from the bottle.

Just for YOU

Are you in recovery from alcohol abuse? The potential benefit your heart receives from alcohol is NOT worth the cost. Don't tell yourself that you can stick with just one drink a day. You can't. Whether you've gone a day or a decade without a drink, alcoholism is a disease for which the only cure is abstinence. Talk with your doctor about other ways to lower your risk of heart disease.

Cardio Care

If a drink a day is your pattern, watch the weight gain. Remember, alcohol's calories are nutritionally empty. Your body converts them to fat almost immediately. One glass of wine a day can add up to an extra 10 pounds a year without physical activity to counteract those added calories. Among the inhibitions alcohol relieves is food intake, adding still more calories.

7. Uh, oh. Red and blue flashing lights. I'd better...

    A. Pull over and get out my license.

    B. Pull over and pretend I'm just getting out of the way.

    C. Roll down the windows, turn the air on full-blast, and pop a roll of breath mints.

    D. Practice touching my nose with my finger.

8. I'm tired of going to family holiday get-togethers. All my relatives ever do is...

    A. Gossip.

    B. Stay up late playing cards.

    C. Tease me about drinking martinis. All they want to do is guzzle beer, and my tastes are more sophisticated.

    D. Nag me about my drinking. I'm an adult, and *I* decide how much is enough for me.

Tally your responses:

As _____   Bs _____   Cs _____   Ds _____

Your highest numbers should be As and Bs. If you have three or more Cs, you're walking the line. All your friends are drinking buddies, and you're starting to hide your drinking. You might benefit from counseling to help you identify and resolve your reasons for drinking (like stress; insecurity; loneliness; and strong emotions like grief, anger, or depression). And if you have any Ds, right now your heart is the least of your problems. You need help to stop drinking before it stops you.

Learning to Ease Up on Alcohol

Cutting down or giving up alcohol isn't easy. Drinking's part of nearly every social event and even takes center stage in some. If you have two or more "D" responses to your self-quiz, start your efforts with a visit to your doctor. The odds are high that you have a physical dependence on alcohol that may need medical assistance to break. If you feel you just drink too much as a pattern of behavior you've slipped into, here are three tips to replace drinking with more healthful activities:

➤ **Break out of your ruts.** Do you go out every Friday night to the same places with the same people? If you usually go for beer and darts, try something where alcohol's not so prominent and the activity level's higher. It's hard to drink when you're moving.

➤ **Find friends who can support your efforts to reduce or stop drinking.** What do you have in common with your current friends besides drinking? What would you do or talk about if you weren't drinking? If you don't know, it's time to move on.

➤ **When you do drink, eat.** Food both slows your body's absorption of alcohol and keeps your mouth and hands busy. Drinking becomes part of another activity, not an activity of its own. Of course, moderation matters here, too. You want to drink less, not eat more!

This Is Your Heart on Drugs

Drugs hide behind many masks. Some we don't even think of as drugs, like cigarettes (nicotine) and alcohol. Others make us feel better when we're sick, like cold medications and antacids. Some we get from the doctor, and some are illegal. All affect your heart.

Happy, healthy substance abusers? Don't bet your life on it. Substances that alter your consciousness change your body. The more often and longer you use these substances, the more damage they do.

The Extraordinary Danger of Cocaine

No hedging on this point: The first time you use cocaine could be your last. Cocaine can cause sudden cardiac death, a steep price for a 20-minute high. Professional basketball will never forget the loss of standout talent Len Bias, who died of a heart attack within hours of using cocaine for the first time. The Boston Celtics had just named the 22-year-old their number-two draft pick in the 1986 pro basketball draft, and Bias and some friends were celebrating.

Though cocaine has a reputation as the recreational drug of choice among the young, nearly half of all emergency room visits for cocaine-related problems involve adults over age 35. Cocaine appears to cause ventricular *tachycardia* (rapid beating) and *fibrillation* (fluttering), robbing your heart of its ability to pump blood out to your body. Doctors can't use the most common emergency room treatment for these conditions, intravenous injection of lidocaine. Chemically, cocaine and lidocaine are too much alike—giving lidocaine makes the situation worse. Cocaine-related heart attacks are nearly always fatal.

Take It to Heart

Cocaine comes from the leaves of the coca plant, which grows in South America. Ancient Inca surgeons had their patients chew coca leaves before undergoing procedures like setting broken bones and removing bone fragments from war wounds. Today, cocaine has legitimate, albeit limited, medical use. Surgeons sometimes spray or swab a mild cocaine solution inside the nose before minor nose surgery. This shrinks blood vessels close to the surface (which reduces bleeding) and numbs the tissue. The drug's action is very fast and lasts for about an hour. Because of cocaine's high abuse potential, however, many doctors prefer to use other anesthetic drugs instead.

When Your Heart Can't Stand the Pain

Red Alert!
Illicit injected drugs carry a risk of bacterial endocarditis, or heart valve infections. Bacteria can enter your bloodstream at the point of injection, particularly if you use dirty needles or don't clean your skin with alcohol. Endocarditis can threaten your life or leave you with permanent damage to your heart valves. Treatment usually involves hospitalization for high doses of intravenous antibiotics.

So what's an aching heart to do? Often, just limp along until something gives—your liver, maybe, or your brain. Occasionally, the pain's more than your heart can bear, and it gives. Here's a sampling of what can happen:

➤ **Amphetamines**, which stimulate your brain and nervous system, can also raise your blood pressure.

➤ **Narcotics**, like codeine and meperidine, slow your heart rate.

➤ **Cocaine** can cause your coronary arteries to spasm and can interfere with your heart's electrical impulses.

➤ **Hallucinogens**, like LSD, mescaline, and psilocybin mushrooms, cause high blood pressure and rapid heart rate.

➤ **Marijuana** smoke interferes with oxygen exchange in your lungs, reducing the amount of oxygen that gets into your bloodstream and to your heart.

Getting Help

Many illicit drugs are highly addictive—your body "needs" them. Even when you want to stop, your body won't let you. Get help. You don't have to go it alone—and you'll be more successful at quitting when you have professionals to guide you and answer your questions. Most health insurance plans provide some sort of coverage for substance-abuse treatment. Your local public health department can also provide help, either through programs it operates or by referring you to qualified programs in your community. And of course, your doctor is always a good place to start.

Your Daily Doses

What drugs do you take every day? Not those your doctor prescribes, but those in the foods and drinks you consume. We've talked in other chapters about the vitamins, minerals, and other substances in certain foods that help you maintain heart health. Here, we're talking about other chemicals that counteract those efforts—ones you sometimes don't even know you're ingesting. (If you smoke, add nicotine, which we discuss in Chapter 21, "Light Up Your Heart, Not a Cigarette" to your list.)

Take It to Heart

Caffeine has long been used as a treatment for headaches, particularly migraines. Some pain medications still include caffeine. Ironically, caffeine can also cause headaches in people who regularly consume moderate to large amounts of caffeine (especially more than five cups of coffee a day) and miss a "dose" or cut back their intake.

Caffeine Keeps the Day Going

Ah, nothing like the smell and taste of java in the morning to get you up and going. You're not alone in your daily pick-me-up. Eight out of ten American adults drink at least one cup of coffee a day. You might feel like the busy lifestyle that gives coffee such status is a phenomenon of the technology age. But coffee's been around since at least A.D. 500, when ancient cultures used coffee beans as currency. No bother with brewing back then—folks just chewed a few beans. Coffee's not the only source of caffeine. Tea, chocolate, and cola drinks all contain caffeine. So do some nonprescription pain medications.

Caffeine is a mild stimulant, and it causes your blood vessels to dilate (get bigger). Too much caffeine can cause *palpitations*, frightening but usually harmless sensations that your heart momentarily stops, then flutters. While palpitations can indicate a rhythm problem with your heart, caffeine-related palpitations go away as soon as the level of caffeine in your body drops (about two hours after your last "dose"). If your palpitations don't go away, schedule an appointment with your doctor.

Red Alert!
Trying to sober someone up? Hot coffee, and the caffeine it contains, is no substitute for the only thing that really works: Time. A drunk who seems more alert after a few cups of coffee may well be, but is no less intoxicated.

Do you consume caffeine to cram more into each day than it's designed to hold? Odds are, you don't have time for other events the day should hold, either, like nutritious meals and regular exercise. This substitution is far more hazardous to your heart health than caffeine.

What's in Your Medicine Cabinet?

Been a while since you've gone through all those half-empty bottles and opened boxes? Time for a cleaning day! First, throw away everything that's past its expiration date by flushing it down the drain. (Check the label; if you don't find an expiration date, trash the product.)

OK. Now take a close look at what's left. Start reading the labels. How many carry the warning, "Do not take this product if you have high blood pressure or heart disease?"

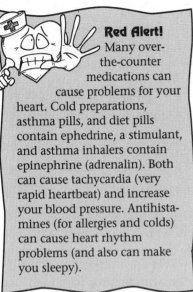

Red Alert! Many over-the-counter medications can cause problems for your heart. Cold preparations, asthma pills, and diet pills contain ephedrine, a stimulant, and asthma inhalers contain epinephrine (adrenalin). Both can cause tachycardia (very rapid heartbeat) and increase your blood pressure. Antihistamines (for allergies and colds) can cause heart rhythm problems (and also can make you sleepy).

Red Alert! Alcohol and acetaminophen, the main ingredient in Tylenol, is an especially dangerous mix. Both drugs affect your liver and, in combination, can send you into liver failure.

These contain ingredients that can speed your heart rate and constrict your blood vessels, causing your blood pressure to rise. If you have either condition, talk to your doctor or pharmacist before using these products. (Pay attention to other "Do not take" warnings, too.)

Deadly Combinations

Mixing medications can produce deadly combinations. Even substances as seemingly innocent as antacids and laxatives can cause potentially fatal magnesium poisoning. Do you take prescription medicines? Ask your pharmacist if there are over-the-counter products you should avoid. Some combinations can make either or both drugs less or more effective, with unpredictable and undesirable results.

Taking illicit drugs is risky enough, since street drugs are of unpredictable purity and can contain a number of hazardous "fillers." But combining them with each other or with alcohol can be a recipe for death. High-profile casualties of drug-related heart attacks include actors John Belushi, River Phoenix, and Chris Farley.

100% Pure Heart

So why use these substances, anyway? Except for prescription medications for short-term pain control, none of the drugs we've discussed in this chapter is something you just can't live without. Stay alert by getting enough sleep, eating nutritious foods, and taking a brisk walk when you feel tired. Relax and relieve stress with meditation, yoga, or martial arts. Come clean! Your heart will love it—and so will you.

The Least You Need to Know

➤ Most doctors agree that more research is necessary before we can credit alcohol with saving hearts.

➤ The first time you use cocaine could be your last. Cocaine can cause sudden cardiac death.

➤ Mixing drugs—over-the-counter, prescription, or illicit—is dangerous. Especially don't combine anything with alcohol.

➤ Getting plenty of exercise and eating right are the best natural highs for a healthy heart.

Part 6
Putting Your Heart in the Right Place

"Once I had brains, and a heart also; so having tried them both, I should much rather have a heart."

—*The Tin Woodsman in* The Wonderful Wizard of Oz.

In some ways, the quest for heart health is like a trip to Oz. You search and search, survive challenges of all sorts, then discover you've had what you're looking for all along. Your heart's not asking you for anything you don't have or can't give. Your heart just wants you to listen to its messages and follow its lead.

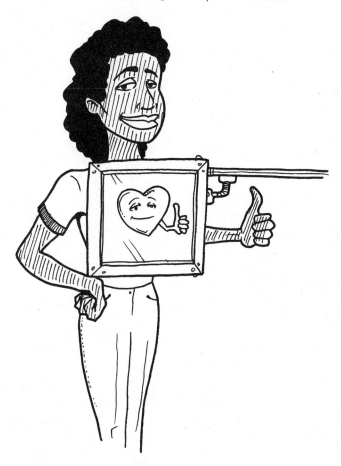

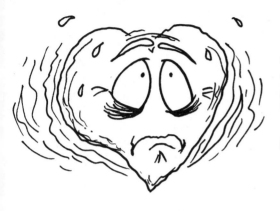

Stress: What to Do When Life's a Blur

While much of heart health is physical (diet and exercise), your mental state plays a role, too. The way you handle stress could explain why, in the absence of other risk factors for heart disease, you have a heart attack—when the guy next door who sits in his chaise lounge with a bag of chips, waving to you as you jog by his house, does not.

You're at greater risk for a heart attack during times of stress, such as during a divorce or after losing a job. Heart attacks are also more common during a crisis. Heart attack rates go up during earthquakes, hurricanes, and other natural disasters. Heart attacks are also more common during the Christmas holiday season. Times of high stress, it seems, are times of high risk for your heart.

What Does Stress Have to Do with My Heart?

Just for YOU
Social expectations about how women behave have created a presentation of "type A" behavior unique to women. While "type A" women certainly can display the more common male "type A" behaviors of hostility, anger, and aggression, "type A" women are more likely to appear very anxious and overly accommodating of the needs of others, and are less likely to express anger. "Type A" women are four times more likely to develop heart disease than are their "type B" counterparts, a risk twice that of "type A" men.

In the 1960s, researchers noticed that impatient, hard-driving, ambitious men had more heart attacks than did their colleagues who were easy-going, casual, and unrushed. They labeled the first group a "type A" personality and the second group "type B." Studies since then show that people with "type A" personalities have high levels of stress hormones in their bodies for long periods of time. While people with "type B" personalities experience spikes of stress hormones related to specific events throughout the day, their levels quickly return to normal.

Researchers don't fully understand the relationship between stress hormones and heart disease. They do know that signs of "type A" personality can show up in young children and that "type A" behaviors in college students are a good indicator for early heart disease in adulthood. Half of American men and a third of American women fit "type A" personality profiles.

What's Your Type?

Go through the following lists, and check the characteristics that apply to you to see whether your personality puts you at risk for heart disease. While many people have traits of both personality types, if yours is predominantly "A," it's time for some stress reduction.

Type A		Type B	
____	Never late, irritated with those who are	____	Not particularly pressured by appointments
____	Highly competitive, every-man-for-himself approach	____	Team-oriented, for-the-common-good approach
____	Frequently interrupt, finish sentences for others	____	Listen attentively, wait until speaker finishes before responding
____	Always have many irons in the fire	____	Do things one at a time
____	Hate to wait, find fault, complain to others who are also waiting	____	Read, think, talk with others while waiting

Type A		Type B	
____	Rush to get work done by its deadline	____	Plan workload to finish by its deadline
____	Gesture, wave hands, pound desk or table when talking	____	Let words carry the conversation
____	Never any doubt about your mood or feelings	____	Mood stays fairly steady, don't show feelings
____	Extrinsically motivated (need outside recognition)	____	Intrinsically motivated (motivated from within)
____	Work is main interest	____	Work is one of many interests

Five Myths About Stress

"The trouble with people is not that they don't know, but that they know so much that ain't so," said 19th-century wit Josh Billings. What do you know about stress? Here are five common myths:

➤ **Myth:** There's no such thing as "good" stress.

Fact: Without some stress, life would be pretty dull. A healthy level of stress provides motivation and stimulation. Stress becomes a problem when it becomes the rule rather than the exception.

➤ **Myth:** Stress is all in your head.

Fact: Stress has a number of direct physical effects. One is that it increases *catecholamine* levels in your blood (biochemical substances your body releases in response to stress). Catecholamines may reduce the flow of blood to your heart. Their levels also go up when you have a heart attack. On the flip side of this matter, physical illness creates a tremendous amount of emotional stress.

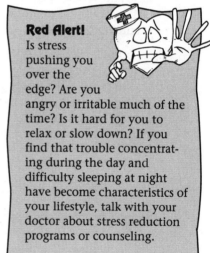

Red Alert!
Is stress pushing you over the edge? Are you angry or irritable much of the time? Is it hard for you to relax or slow down? If you find that trouble concentrating during the day and difficulty sleeping at night have become characteristics of your lifestyle, talk with your doctor about stress reduction programs or counseling.

➤ **Myth:** We live in stressful times. There's nothing you can do about that.

Fact: While our culture seems filled with stressful events, there's plenty you can do to reduce the ways these events affect you. A big portion of stress is not so much the event as the way you view it. Can you change the situation causing you stress? If so, do it. If not, change your attitude about it, and the event becomes less stressful.

➤ **Myth:** Stress keeps you sharp, focused, and organized.

Fact: It might in the short term, but a little stress goes a long way. Continuous or frequent stress appears to numb your body's responses, though, having the opposite effect. Too much stress causes fragmented thinking and inability to act.

➤ **Myth:** If you don't feel stressed out, you don't need to worry about stress reduction techniques.

Fact: Stress affects your body and your mind, whether you're aware of it or not. Continued exposure to high levels of stress numbs your perceptions of stress responses. Your perception that your life is stress-free may instead be a strong sign that you've reached stress overload. Regularly practicing relaxation techniques helps keep your stress levels low.

"But I Like Living on the Edge!"

Do you? Or are you just so used to it that you don't know any other way to live? It can be quite a rush, living in a state of continual crisis. It's also an interesting study for psychologists and cardiologists alike! As much as you might like living on the edge, your body's not especially fond of the habit. It's always "on alert," at the ready to fight or flee. (Remember fight or flight?)

Your body responds to the signals of stress by gearing up, it mistakenly thinks, to save your life. Your heart rate quickens, your blood pressure surges, and your senses heighten. You're powered to throw your spear straight and true, right into the eye of that tiger... or race like the wind back to your cave. Wait a minute. What's wrong with this picture? Spear? Cave? Tiger? Are these elements of your typical day? Of course not. But your pressured, stressful life activates these primordial responses just the same. As a result, your body's engine—your heart—runs in constant overdrive. It doesn't take you any farther, it just works harder to get you where you're going. At some point, all that extra work will wear it down.

Living in the Moment: Cultivating Mindfulness

What's happening within you right now? Not around you, but within you, in your body and in your mind. If you really don't know, don't worry—most of us are not very mindful much of the time. Though if we were, we'd have far less stress in our lives. Mindfulness is the experience of being aware of the moment.

Jon Kabat-Zinn, Ph.D., who directs the Stress Reduction Clinic at the University of Massachusetts Medical Center, likens mindfulness to thinking of your mind as an ocean. You notice that there are big waves and small waves, observe each as it forms, rolls in toward the beach, and breaks. Your mission is not to flatten the waves into smooth calmness, but to learn how to surf. You see each wave clearly, says Kabat-Zinn, and simply ride it to shore.

Mindfulness, then, is like "thought-surfing." This shifts your emphasis from worrying about what might happen to what is happening, which is often a far smaller matter. The result is less focus on the details of life that drive you crazy, because you're not trying to control anything. You simply see and accept.

The Fine Art of Meditation

What image comes to your mind when you think of meditation? Many people view meditation as an Eastern religion of sorts, something only those well-practiced in stringent self-discipline can do. While meditation is an aspect of many Eastern belief systems, rather like prayer is an element of many Western belief systems, it's not itself a religion. Anyone can meditate, and everyone who does benefits.

By Heart
Meditation comes from the Latin word *meditari*, which means "remedy." While common perception is that meditation is a process of deep thinking, it's actually a means of focusing your mind to reduce or eliminate conscious thought, to bring your mind to stillness or rest.

Meditation allows you to go inside yourself. Some forms of meditation involve focusing on one thing to the exclusion of all others. You might, for example, sit comfortably and close your eyes, then focus entirely on the process of breathing. Anything else that enters your mind, you deliberately and consciously push aside until all that remains is your awareness of your breathing. The process leaves your mind refreshed and invigorated. Other forms of meditation may incorporate guided imagery techniques or mindfulness.

"The Hurrieder I Go, the Behinder I Get"

A poster bearing this homespun observation made by baseball legend and folk philosopher Satchel Paige hangs on the wall of a busy dental office. A dozen staff bustle here and there as the waiting room runs out of chairs. Clearly, they've missed the point. The only way to do more is to slow down. Yet many of us seem addicted to time. We rush around, though we're always late. In his book *Slow Down... and Get More Done*, Marshall J. Cook calls this malady of modern culture "speed sickness." Do you have speed sickness? If so, it's taking you nowhere fast. Call a time-out! Sit down, catch your breath. You don't gain any more time trying to do more with less. You just get frustrated, angry, and tense, which takes you back to fight-or-flight.

Just for YOU
Studies show that women with metastatic breast cancer who join support groups live twice as long as women who don't. Scientists in the field of psychoneuroimmunology believe the sharing and interaction that takes place in such groups reduce stress, which in turn boosts the immune system.

245

The Mind/Body Connection

It's really a perception of Western culture that the body and mind are separate. Much of the world views human existence in a more unified, holistic way that integrates body and mind (and spirit or soul) into a single, inseparable being. Western medicine is coming to accept a similar view as an increasing body of research reveals more about what emotions and feelings do to the brain.

Some researchers believe that emotions are actually the bridge that links the body and the mind. One is Candace Pert, Ph.D., the molecular biologist who discovered the presence and role of *endorphins* and *neuropeptides*. These biochemical substances interact with receptors within your body's cells. This research has far-reaching implications for many health problems, including heart disease. Doctors have long known that there is a connection between anger and heart attacks, for example, though they haven't known what exactly the connection is. Neuropeptides may provide the explanation, as well as a means of breaking the link.

Biofeedback: Body Talk

"It's OK to talk to yourself," goes the old saying, "as long as you don't talk back." *Biofeedback* is more like talking to yourself, then listening to what your body says back. Many people use biofeedback techniques to relieve muscle tension and pain from conditions like migraine headaches. Biofeedback can be as simple as training yourself to become aware of how tense your muscles are (as a clue to your stress level), then using relaxation techniques to untense them (and reduce stress). With extensive training and practice, some people have had success using biofeedback to lower blood pressure (don't try this yourself without your doctor's permission, especially if you're taking medication for high blood pressure).

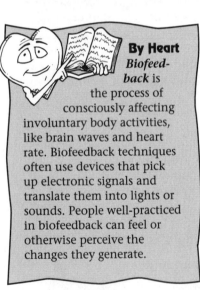

Cardio Care
If you think biofeedback might help you lower your blood pressure, ask your doctor for a referral to a qualified biofeedback clinic. While eventually biofeedback will become a technique you can practice on your own, you need proper training to learn what to do and how to do it. Don't stop taking blood pressure medication until your doctor says it's safe for you to do so.

By Heart
Biofeedback is the process of consciously affecting involuntary body activities, like brain waves and heart rate. Biofeedback techniques often use devices that pick up electronic signals and translate them into lights or sounds. People well-practiced in biofeedback can feel or otherwise perceive the changes they generate.

Guided Imagery: See the Life You Want

Imagine, for a moment, that you're in a forest. It's quiet and peaceful, and you feel safe and comfortable. Imagine yourself walking through this forest, stepping softly on a path covered with thick moss. You hear the leaves rustling in a gentle breeze, smell a hint of water. You reach a small stream. Put your fingers in the water, feel its refreshing coolness against your skin. Sit on that rounded rock at the water's edge, and pull off your shoes and socks. Slip your feet into the water, furrow your toes into the sandy bottom. Relaxing, isn't it? A lovely break from the stress and worry of your busy day, and you haven't even left your living room or desk or wherever you're sitting right now.

You can take yourself on such a journey anytime, no matter where you are (though we don't recommend you try this while driving). It's called *guided imagery,* and it's a powerful tool for both stress reduction and healing. Some people use (and doctors recommend) guided imagery to envision recovery and health. You can imagine anything you want. Feel free to let your spiritual or religious beliefs become part of your guided-imagery experience. What's most important is that you feel safe and protected, and that you visualize healing and happiness. What that looks like is up to you.

Spirituality: Soul Support

Do you go to church regularly? Studies show that what's good for the soul is also good for the body. You're more likely to survive serious illness or injury, including heart surgery, if you go to church regularly. It doesn't matter what religion, denomination, or belief system you practice. Spirituality benefits your physical health because it helps you move beyond your personal difficulties. Churches also offer a strong community-support network that often includes support groups and social activities. Simply getting involved with a group, even just in social activities, can help you reduce the stress in your life.

Take It to Heart

Does it seem that you do more and enjoy less these days? A movement to simplify life has taken hold across the United States. Supporters say that less is indeed more—the less cluttered you make your life, the more time you have to enjoy what matters. Many of our daily "must-do" activities are self-imposed. Every nonessential task takes time that you could instead spend with your family or doing things for yourself. How much could you simplify your life, and how much would doing so reduce your daily stress level?

Flow: Boost Peak Performance

Musicians call it being "in the groove." Athletes call it being "in the zone." Whatever you call it, it's that point of oneness with yourself when your body, mind, and spirit reach complete balance. It's a wonderful place to be. When you're there, you're on, you're hot, you're infallible. Words, actions, and thoughts flow effortlessly.

So how do you get there? Not by simply willing or commanding yourself. In fact, concentrating on achieving "flow" actually prevents you from reaching it. It's a little like those pictures that, when you first look at them, appear to be nothing more than a collection of shapes and colors. But when you look into them, past the surface of the picture, and relax the focus of your eyes, a three-dimensional image emerges. With enough practice, you can train your eyes to immediately shift to this altered focus as soon as you see one of these pictures, and move right to the image. You can train your body and mind to shift focus in a similar way, to see beyond individual elements to the image beyond. Really, what you're doing is transcending the obvious or the immediate—the surface of the picture, and the surface of your mind and body. Meditation, yoga, and tai chi are useful tools for doing this.

Taking a Heart-Healthy Look at Your Life

Heart health is more than just diet, or exercise, or genetics, or stress. It's the way all these elements come together in your life. Remember homeostasis, the process by which your body systems compensate to restore balance? There's a homeostasis that involves your whole being, too, that achieves balance among your body, mind, and spirit. It's that overall result that accounts for the health of your heart… and the rest of you.

The Least You Need to Know

➤ Not all stress is bad. Stress becomes a problem when it's the rule rather than the exception.

➤ "Type A" personality traits increase your risk for heart disease and heart attack.

➤ Relaxation techniques that reduce stress have measurable physical effects on your body, from lowered blood pressure and heart rate to decreased muscle tension.

➤ The faster you go, the less you accomplish.

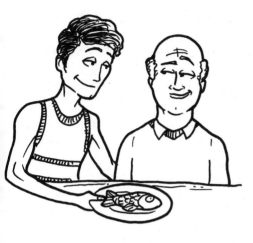

Chapter 24

When Someone You Love Has Heart Trouble

In This Chapter

➤ Choosing the right time and place to talk

➤ Encouraging a loved one to see a doctor

➤ How to handle your own fears and worries

➤ Reentering life

Sometimes the heart problems that trouble you the most are not yours but those of someone you love. And sometimes this is more of a problem than if the heart disease were yours, because you can't change someone else's actions and behaviors.

Having a Heart to Heart

"You fool! Can't you see you're living your way to an early grave?!?" That's what you want to scream when someone you love ignores the obvious. But that's what you *can't* say, if you want your words to have any effect on that special someone's actions. The only way your words will make a difference is if you deliver them with caring and compassion. Here are a few tips to help you say what's in your heart:

➤ **Plan what you'll say.** What worries you about your loved one's actions or situation? Sometimes it helps to write your thoughts out. This focuses your thinking.

➤ **Choose a time when you can talk without interruptions.** Don't go for the time slot of a favorite TV show, a meal, or bedtime. Separate your discussion from other activities. This both gives it importance and removes distractions.

➤ **Make your points clearly and calmly** (refer to your written notes, if that'll help). Try not to be accusing ("You're just too lazy to get your fat butt off the couch!"). Instead, emphasize that love drives your concern ("I want us to watch our grand-children grow up... together").

➤ **Offer to share heart-healthy changes.** No one wants to change alone. It's hard to eat a broiled chicken breast and a salad for lunch when the person across the table's wolfing down a grilled Reuben and big ol' steak fries just oozing grease. (You've gotta wonder why we like this stuff in the first place.) Walk or bicycle together, golf or bowl, or do whatever interests you both.

➤ **Keep the faith.** Even if your first attempt bombs, chances are you've at least made the point that you care. You won't see changes overnight, but you might see bagels replace doughnuts. Remember, the most you can do is support your loved one's changes. You can't make them for him or her.

Take It to Heart

You might think you're too old for peer pressure. After all, you've been an adult for more years than you care to count, maybe raised a family and today enjoy grandchildren. How can others possibly pressure you now? We human beings are social creatures, and what others think and do influences more than we might know. From the cars we drive to the food we eat, the opinions of others shape our choices. The power of this phenomenon was no surprise to British researchers who concluded that heart-healthy lifestyle changes were most consistent and significant in married couples when both partners imple-mented them as shared activities.

Getting Someone You Love to See a Doctor

Many people, particularly those over 60, take great pride in never going to the doctor. "I can take care of myself," they scoff. "Those doctors are just kids, anyway. What do they know about life?" However short on life experience younger doctors may appear to be, they know an awful lot about what it takes to keep you among the living. Today's physi-cians come out of medical school cram-packed with more knowledge than even existed 50 years ago. (Remember, antibiotics, immunizations, and clot busters are all advances of the last half of the 20th century.) And face it—if you're 60 or older, many people are younger than you! But you already know these things, because you see your doctor regularly. It's a spouse, child, sibling, or dear friend who resists.

Why Your Loved One Won't Go to the Doctor: The Excuses

So why does the one you love (who could be you) hate to go to the doctor? Here are some common excuses... check all that apply to your loved one:

❑ You go in for a hangnail, and before you know it, you're having heart surgery.

❑ What I don't know won't hurt me.

❑ My day's so full now, I barely have time to blow my nose. Where am I gonna find time to sit in a doctor's office all afternoon?

❑ Doctors are for sick people. I'll go when I'm sick.

❑ Why should I pay good money to go have a complete stranger tell me what's wrong with me? I've got enough grief in my life already!

❑ I'll go as soon as I lose a few pounds. I don't want my doctor to see me so fat.

❑ I always get a gown with missing ties.

❑ My granddad never missed a day of work and lived to 103. Longevity runs in my family, not heart disease.

❑ "Less fat, more exercise." Easy for them to say!

❑ When it's my time to go, it's my time to go. No doctor's gonna change that.

"So What Can I Do?"

If doctors had the answer for this one, there'd be very little heart disease! Sometimes, you can schedule an appointment and say, "You're going." Beware, that approach can backfire, though. A person who refuses to confront the reality of a heart-threatening lifestyle isn't likely to be terribly forthcoming with the doctor. The visit can end up a frustration for everyone, leaving your loved one more firmly resolved than before to "do it my way." Sometimes, unfortunately, you can't do anything about someone else's dangerous decisions. As adults, we're all entitled to make choices about how we live—even if our decisions doom us to early death. But sometimes you can convince the one you love that life without him or her is a prospect you can't bear to think about. And you can make heart-healthy changes in your own life and hope that your loved one follows your lead.

Take It to Heart

While you might feel like you're the only person in the world who's struggling to cope with a loved one's heart disease, you're far from alone. More than 57 million Americans (10 million of them women) live with heart disease—and so do their families.

Coping with Your Own Fears and Feelings

It's normal to experience a wide range of emotions when someone you love has a heart attack or heart surgery. After all, you've nearly lost the person who fills your life with joy and happiness. You might tumble through fear, anger, denial, panic, sadness, and relief—all in the few minutes it takes for the doctor to explain what's happened. It's a wakeup call for you, too, a reminder of how fragile life is. And even though you're not the one with heart disease, your life changes forever as well. But this isn't necessarily a bad thing! Many changes that your loved one needs to make are for the better... for both of you, if you let them.

Just for YOU
Are you a woman suddenly facing the full responsibility of managing household finances? Classes are available in many communities, often through senior centers and community colleges, to give you a jumpstart in learning what to do and how to do it. Your insurance agent, accountant, bank, or library can often tell you where to find such classes. You might also contact the social services department at the hospital for guidance.

By Heart
Cardiac rehabilitation programs, sometimes called *heart rehab* for short, help you integrate necessary diet and exercise changes into your lifestyle. The program staff has special training in heart conditioning, and many are physical or occupational therapists. Particularly right after you go home from the hospital, your rehab program may include physical therapy to help you get moving again.

Staying with the Treatment Plan

So your loved one went to the doctor, who confirmed your suspicions of heart disease. Or had a heart attack, proof even he or she can't argue with. Now what? In all likelihood, it's time for a major overhaul. Your loved one's probably taking medication, at least for the time being, and possibly for the duration. No more fooling around with fat, no more watching other people work their way through the fitness stations at the park. This is where the rubber hits the road. Unfortunately, it's also where many people skid back to old habits. Try to get those old habits out of the house. Here are some tips to help your transition:

➤ Fill your refrigerator with fruits and vegetables. Replace high-fat favorites in your cupboard with low-fat substitutes. Swap fried chips for baked crackers, and chocolate chip cookies for lower fat oatmeal-raisin cookies (check the labels to be sure you're ditching both fat and calories). Trade cinnamon rolls for cinnamon-raisin bagels.

➤ Invest in a good low-fat cookbook or two. Often, your loved one's doctor can recommend ones that other patients have liked. Or ask at the library or bookstore which ones are popular.

➤ Find ways to make physical activity part of the regular day for both of you (within the limits of your loved one's capabilities). Walk the dog, take the stairs, walk to get the mail.

➤ Make a place and establish a routine for medications, so your loved one has less trouble remembering to take them at the right times.

➤ If you smoke, give it up.

Safety in Numbers

If your loved one has had a heart attack or heart surgery, his or her doctor probably recommended a *cardiac rehabilitation program* to get the new heart-healthy lifestyle off on the right foot. Many such programs encourage significant others to participate in the educational aspects, to learn what changes to make and how to make them. Some programs are available through medical centers, and others through special offerings at places like the YMCA.

Consider joining a fitness club when the rehabilitation program is finished to maintain the good habits your loved one has developed. And sometimes support groups are helpful, too. No matter how much you love someone, you can't know what they're feeling and experiencing unless you've gone through it, too. Support groups offer a chance to share common concerns. There are also support groups for family members and friends to help them share their worries.

Make heart-healthy changes a way of life for everyone in the household. It's hard to be the odd one out, whichever side of the heart-healthy path you're on.

Returning to Social Activities

Sometimes it's hard to get back into the swing of things, particularly if rehabilitation has been long and slow. But getting back is important. It reestablishes your connections to friends and relatives. The "old" life wasn't all bad, and there's no reason to think you have to abandon it entirely. Venturing out into the "real" world can be frightening. Even though others mean well when they express their care and concern, the attention can be uncomfortable. People who are further removed from your life than immediate family and close friends might not understand all that your loved one has been through. Though they mean well, they might ask prying questions or make insensitive comments, especially at first. Spare your loved one by redirecting the conversation to less-intrusive topics. Their lifestyles may be the same as always, which could be incompatible with your heart-healthy one.

Cardio Care
Someone recovering from a heart attack or heart surgery often needs help with everyday activities that were once matter-of-fact. Accepting such help is often more difficult than offering it, however, since we all value our independence. Try an indirect approach—for example, place daily use items within easy reach, put medicines out with meals, or open doors.

Red Alert!
Check with your doctor before entering any heart-health program. Different programs emphasize different things, and you want to find one that's a good match for your needs and capabilities. The wrong program could do more harm than good.

253

Cardio Care
Heading off on a day trip? Stop every hour or so and walk around for 10 to 15 minutes to stretch your legs and invigorate your heart. Plan a picnic and take your own heart-healthy food. Not only will your heart thank you, but you may end up having more fun than if you had to worry about choosing the lesser of two evils from a diner's limited menu.

Red Alert!
Depression is more than a bad case of the blues. Depression can be a serious condition that requires treatment from your doctor and a therapist. Common signs of depression include disinterest in life, problems with sleep (too much or too little), deep sadness, lack of energy, anxiousness, change in appetite, and sometimes irrational anger or hostility.

You can help your loved one make wise decisions by making them yourself. Off to the company picnic? Go for a grilled burger with ketchup and mustard rather than a hotdog, or choose chicken. Try salads instead of mayonnaise-laden potato and macaroni salads. Many catered events present a variety of foods to meet different tastes and needs. If you're going to a potluck event, take a low-fat dish or two so you're guaranteed of at least those choices.

Taking Good Care

Remember to take care of yourself. For obvious reasons, the person with heart trouble takes center stage. This doesn't mean that your well-being is any less important, though. In fact, it may be more important if you now have to step into a leadership role in your household. Get enough rest. Plan time for yourself, time to unwind and deal with your feelings. One of the hard things about dealing with someone else's life-threatening condition is that you can't talk to him or her about your fears and worries—your loved one's pretty preoccupied with his or her brush with mortality.

Consider joining a support group to help yourself work through your concerns. Others in the support group are in varying stages of experiences similar to yours. It's a good opportunity to talk about your feelings and learn how others cope with theirs. If you feel significant stress because of a loved one's health problems, a counselor can help you sort through your feelings and find ways to manage your concerns. Remember, major stresses in your life (such as a new job, retirement, divorce, health problems, or death of a loved one) can trigger depression.

The Least You Need to Know

➤ A loved one's heart attack, heart surgery, or heart disease means changes in your life, too.

➤ It's normal and OK to feel frightened, angry, sad, and frustrated about a loved one's heart trouble. It helps to talk about your fears and worries with a friend who knows you both.

➤ You don't have to throw out everything from the "old" life to live a heart-healthy lifestyle.

➤ Make heart-healthy living a change for your entire household. Everyone, including your loved one, will benefit.

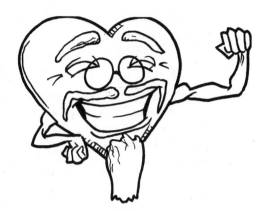

Chapter 25

A Light Heart Lives Long

In This Chapter

➤ You've got what it takes

➤ How to listen to your heart

➤ How happy is your heart: A self-quiz

➤ The heart-healthy way to a long life

Even though they didn't quite get the details right, ancient healers were on the right track when they identified the heart as the center of existence. And they were right on target when they recognized the importance of considering the whole being—body, mind, and soul—when it came to the success of medical treatment. "...as you ought not to attempt to cure the eyes without the head, or the head without the body, so neither ought you attempt to cure the body without the soul... for the part can never be well until the whole is well," wrote the philosopher Plato.

Your heart sets the rhythm of your life. The lifestyle choices you make help keep that beat strong and steady, helping it to carry you through a long and happy life.

Oz Never Did Give Nothin' to the Tin Man

In the fantasy story that's delighted millions of readers since its publication in 1900, L. Frank Baum's *The Wonderful Wizard of Oz*, the Tin Woodman journeys to the magical land of Oz seeking what he thinks he's missing—a heart. As it turns out, what he so desperately sought was already within him. He had more than enough heart, he just didn't recognize it. Like the Tin Woodman, you've already got what you need for heart health and happiness—all you have to do is recognize it and use it.

Listening to Your Heart

We've talked throughout this book about the messages your heart sends you. But have you ever listened to your heart, actually heard it beating within you? Take a few moments right now to try it. Just sit, still and calm, close your eyes if that helps you focus, and listen for your heartbeat. The sounds you're trying to hear are soft and almost muffled compared to the ones you'd hear through a stethoscope. These sounds you're listening for now reach your eardrums from the inside, unlike the sounds you're used to that bounced in from the outside. Bone is a very good conductor, and it carries the sound of your heartbeat to your eardrums quite well.

Concentrate on shutting out outside noises. If you can't hear your heart beating, don't panic. It's still right there in the center of your chest, pumping life through your body with every lubb-dupp. It can take practice to hear it. But keep trying. Hearing your heart at work is an awesome experience. It's a most clear and vivid reminder that you are alive.

Following Your Heart

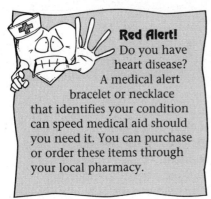

Red Alert!
Do you have heart disease? A medical alert bracelet or necklace that identifies your condition can speed medical aid should you need it. You can purchase or order these items through your local pharmacy.

How would your life change if you let your heart take the lead? You might be among the fortunate few whose habits would change little. Most of us would take a very different path than the one we now travel. Your heart would have you eat when your body signaled its need for nourishment, not at the whiff of a cinnamon roll or whim of a clock. Your legs would take you most places you go, as much as possible. You'd break a good sweat at least four or five times a week, sleep when you were tired, and take more time for yourself than for the details of living. Relaxation techniques would be an automatic response to stress, harmlessly deflecting potential ill effects. So what keeps you from following your heart?

Is Your Heart Really Happy?: A Self-Quiz

Do you give your heart what it desires? Answer these questions (for how you live now, not how you plan to live after reading this book) to find out:

1. I exercise hard enough to break a sweat...

    A. Seven days a week.

    B. Four, sometimes five, days a week.

    C. Fewer than three days a week.

    D. Only on Saturdays.

2. I eat red meat...
   A. Never.
   B. Once or twice a month, I grill or broil a lean cut.
   C. Every Friday night.
   D. With every meal.

3. My favorite relaxation technique is...
   A. A 20-mile run every day.
   B. Meditation or yoga daily.
   C. A walk through the park or on the beach.
   D. A few hours of TV.

4. I fall asleep...
   A. Before my head even hits the pillow. By the end of the day, I'm exhausted.
   B. About 15 minutes or so after I go to bed.
   C. An hour or so after I go to bed. Even though I feel tired, I toss and turn.
   D. Anywhere, any time.

5. I use guided imagery...
   A. Every time I have a few free minutes.
   B. When there are particularly stressful events taking place in my life, including physical illness.
   C. When nothing else works to reduce my stress level.
   D. When I'm lost and I need directions.

6. "Time for myself" means...
   A. Living alone.
   B. Making and keeping dates with myself to do fun things that have no purpose other than enjoyment.
   C. Getting to work an hour earlier than anyone else.
   D. I'm the main attraction.

Just for YOU
Since 1984, women have outnumbered men in dying from heart disease, and the gap continues to widen. Lifestyle choices seem the culprit—smoking, high-fat diet, and a sedentary lifestyle are now common among women (particularly those in the workforce). The risk of heart disease shoots alarmingly high after menopause, as the protective effect of estrogen wanes. Heart-healthy choices early in life may be even more important for women.

Do you have more than four As? You might be trying too hard, which can be nearly as hazardous as not trying hard enough. If you're feeling like your life's more sacrifice than satisfaction, ease up a little. Your body needs rest and relaxation, too. More than four Bs?

You're doing your heart good! More than four Cs? You're on the right track, though not entirely tuned in. Your lifestyle probably needs less stress, less dietary fat, and more regular exercise. More than four Ds? Hope you've been paying attention as you've been reading, especially those sections on how to make heart-healthy changes in your lifestyle.

Opening Your Heart

Cardio Care

If you find it difficult to confide in friends or family members, consider joining a support group or scheduling a few visits with a therapist. In these settings, you can discuss your concerns with others who share them, or who can guide you in dealing with them.

People who talk to other people are happier and live longer than those who don't. Study after study confirms it. Sharing and communicating releases stress. Connections with other people give your life an outside purpose, a reason for being that extends beyond you. For some people, talking comes as naturally as breathing. For others, talking (the kind that requires sharing thoughts and feelings) takes considerable effort.

When you talk about how you feel, you surface worries and fears that otherwise would remain buried deep in your subconscious mind. Since what we fear most is the un-known, your hidden concerns fester, causing stress, until they erupt into physical conditions like digestive distur-bances and headaches—and high blood pressure, strokes, and heart attacks. When you can talk about your fears, they become less frightening—and less stressful.

Take It to Heart

Do you find it hard to listen when someone else is talking? The average person listens at a rate of about 400 words a minute, yet speaks at 80 to 90 words a minute. Your mind finds it distracting to wait all that time for the next word, so it starts doing other things. You might start thinking about what to fix for dinner, what the weather will be like tomorrow, or even what you're going to say once the other person stops talking. To help rein in your wandering mind, maintain eye contact with the other person, and concentrate on other aspects of communication like voice tone and body gestures.

Are you an *introvert* or an *extrovert*? Knowing your general communication style can help you understand why you find it difficult to talk about your concerns... or talk about them all the time. People who process information internally (introverts) often have trouble airing their worries and feelings. But the extra effort is worthwhile; being able to talk about what concerns you helps decrease the frustration that builds when you keep your feelings bottled inside you. People who are outgoing and talkative (extroverts) generally have little difficulty discussing their concerns. Do you and your loved one approach communication differently? Give your loved one the advantage here, and try to accommodate his or her style.

Keep a Young Heart

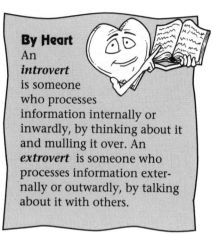

By Heart
An *introvert* is someone who processes information internally or inwardly, by thinking about it and mulling it over. An *extrovert* is someone who processes information externally or outwardly, by talking about it with others.

So what's the point of all this heart-healthy living? Most of us want not only to live longer, but also to live well. The prospect of growing old and infirm has little appeal. Yet who wouldn't look forward to growing old and staying healthy? Remember, where your heart leads, the rest of you follows. Keep your heart young and fit, and it can lead you to a most pleasant rest of your life.

The Secrets of Healthy Aging

It really should come as little surprise to learn that the world's oldest people live in small, often remote communities removed from what we've come to view as the essentials of modern life. Yet they don't feel life has passed them by. They've lived life to the fullest, and their regrets are few. Could they have lived similarly healthy lives in, say, Boston or Seattle, where they had to make the same kinds of difficult choices as you do? Hard to say. But you can. You have the knowledge you need to choose the lifestyle your heart desires, a lifestyle of health and longevity.

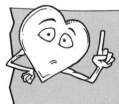

Take It to Heart

According to recent studies, patients who *think* they will be up and around six weeks after a heart attack usually are—and do better overall than patients whose outlooks are less positive.

The Power of Positive Thinking

"Look on the bright side." "Every cloud has its silver lining." "As you think, so you are." These motivational moments are more than just platitudes. They cut right to the heart of healthy living: attitude. Healers have known since the time of Plato that there are powerful connections between your thoughts and your health. "Before you can heal the body, you must heal the mind," the ancient Greek philosopher instructed his followers.

Few dispute the relationship between negative thoughts and bad health outcomes. Yet we often resist the reverse—that positive thoughts influence good health outcomes.

Cardio Care
In his book *Positive Thinking Every Day*, Norman Vincent Peale offers this advice: "Medication is of course important but do not conclude that a pill dissolving in your stomach is necessarily more powerful than a healing thought dissolving in your mind."

Admittedly, when something's wrong, we want to know what, why, and how to fix it. Preventing that "wrong" from happening in the first place is harder to focus on, because it's more difficult to prove. Is the absence of disease evidence enough that a positive attitude improves health? More and more doctors believe so.

Creating a Happy, Heart-Healthy World

It's no longer an impossible dream. Look at the changes just in the last 10 years. Government buildings and many private offices have beanned inside smoking. There's no smoking in airports or on domestic flights. Restaurants feature heart-healthy menu selections (even egg-substitute omelets), and some specialize in them. Even fast-food chains now offer low-fat alternatives. Big business deals are more likely to be brokered in the gym, on the handball court, or on the golf course than in the lounge. Ten thousand people ride their bicycles from Seattle, Washington, to Portland, Oregon, every summer during the nation's largest organized bicycle event. The Boston Marathon draws 12,000 runners from around the world; the New York Marathon entices more than 29,000 participants to pound the pavement. Heart surgery gives nearly five million people a second chance at life each year—many of whom fully recover to run, bicycle, and enjoy many other activities. And people like you are buying books like this to learn more about preventing heart disease in the first place.

The Least You Need to Know

➤ Share your life with people who care about you. It's good for your heart.

➤ You can't always control the events in your life, but you can control your reactions to them. A positive attitude can deflate stress.

➤ Live long, and live healthy. Your heart will lead the way.

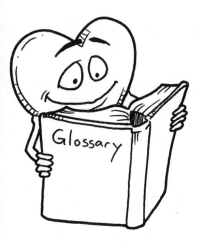

Glossary

ACE inhibitor   A drug that makes the heart's work easier by blocking chemicals that constrict capillaries.

aerobic   Means "in the presence of oxygen." Aerobic exercise causes your heart to beat harder and faster, carrying more oxygen to your hard-at-work muscles.

allopathy   Conventional medicine practiced by physicians who graduate from medical school and write "MD" after their names.

alveoli   The tiny sacs deep within the lungs where the oxygen–carbon dioxide exchange takes place.

anaerobic   Without oxygen.

anemia   A medical condition in which the body lacks sufficient hemoglobin, resulting in reduced oxygen to body tissues.

angina pectoris   Pain in the heart from insufficient oxygen (blood flow) to the heart muscle.

angiography   A test in which dye is injected into an artery to make the actions of the heart and circulatory system visible using moving x-rays.

angioplasty   A procedure in which a balloon-tipped catheter is inserted through a vein and into the blocked portion of a coronary artery to enlarge the narrowing. Also called *percutaneous transluminal coronary angioplasty* (PTCA).

anticoagulant   A drug that prevents clots from forming.

aorta   A large artery through which blood leaves the heart to go to the rest of the body.

"apple" body shape   Extra body weight carried around the waist, a pattern that correlates with a higher risk of heart disease than a "pear" body shape.

arrhythmias   Electrical irregularities in the heart.

artificial heart   A mechanical device to assist a failing heart until a transplant organ can be located.

aspirin therapy   One baby aspirin or one-half adult aspirin tablet taken daily to help prevent clots from forming.

atria   The upper two chambers of the heart.

atrium   One of the heart's two upper chambers.

auscultation   Listening to the heart and lungs using a stethoscope.

beta blocker   A drug that reduces the rate and force of the heart's pumping action to reduce its oxygen needs.

biofeedback   The process of consciously affecting involuntary body activities, like brain waves and heart rate.

blood pressure   The highest and lowest pressures within the arteries that occur during the cardiac cycle. Measured in millimeters of mercury.

bradycardia   A heart rate that is slower than normal.

brain death   The absence of electrical activity in the brain, as measured by an electroencephalograph.

calcium channel blocker   A drug that slows the movement of calcium across the membranes of heart muscle cells to slow their contraction.

cardiac catheterization   A diagnostic procedure during which a small tube, or catheter, is threaded into the arteries around the heart.

cardiac rehabilitation programs   Sometimes called *heart rehab*. Helps you integrate necessary diet and exercise changes into your lifestyle.

cardiologist   A physician who specializes in heart problems.

cardiomyopathy   An enlarged heart that no longer pumps effectively. Some cardiomyopathies have known causes, such as alcholic cardiomyopathy. Many occur for no known reason, and are called *idiopathic*.

cardiovascular   Of the heart and blood vessels.

cardiovascular disease (CVD)   Any of several diseases involving the heart and blood vessels, including high blood pressure, coronary heart disease, stroke, rheumatic heart disease, and other heart and blood vessel problems.

cardioversion   A mild shock delivered to the heart through the chest wall (given in a hospital under light sedation) to redirect the heart to a normal rhythm.

cartoid artery   The artery felt in the neck below the jawbone. Often used for taking the pulse during exercise.

chelation therapy   The technique of introducing a substance into the circulatory system to remove minerals from the body. Often used to treat poisoning by heavy metals like iron, lead, and arsenic. Used experimentally to attempt to reduce arterial plaque.

cholesterol   A chemical called a *lipid* that the body uses to make cell membranes and some hormones. HDL cholesterol, or *high density lipoprotein*, is "good" cholesterol. LDL cholesterol, or *low density lipoprotein*, is "bad" cholesterol.

cloning   The scientific process of producing an exact duplicate of a gene, cell, or organism.

clot busters   Drugs called thrombolytics that rapidly dissolve blood clots, "unplugging" blocked arteries to restore blood flow.

congenital heart disease   A heart problem present from birth.

Coronary artery bypass graft (CABG)   Surgical reconstruction of the arteries supplying the heart.

CT scan   Computerized tomography, a sophisticated diagnostic imaging procedure that uses a computer and x-rays to present cross-section "slices" of areas of the body.

diastole   Means "to dilate" or "to expand." The time during which the heart's chambers relax and fill with blood. The lower number in a blood-pressure reading.

digitalis   A drug that regulates the rate and strength of the heartbeat (digoxin, digi-toxin).

diuretic   A drug that reduces blood volume by increasing the amount of water the kidneys extract as they filter the blood. Sometimes called "water pills."

echocardiography   Ultrasound examination of the heart.

electrocardiogram (ECG, EKG)   A test that produces tracings of the heart's electrical activity. The process of performing an ECG is called *electrocardiography*, which means "electric heart writing."

endorphins   Natural substances, chemically similar to morphine, that the brain releases to relieve pain.

erythrocytes   Red blood cells.

evolution   The process by which plant and animal species change in response to changes in their environments.

expiration   The process by which the lungs expel air; also called *exhalation*.

extrovert   A person who processes information externally or outwardly, by talking about it with others.

familial hyperlipidemia   High cholesterol and triglyceride levels that are genetic or run in the family.

fasting   Refraining from food (and sometimes drink). Certain tests or procedures may require 12 to 14 hours of fasting before they can be accurately performed.

fibrillation   Very rapid, disorganized beating of the heart.

food pyramid   A chart, drawn in the shape of a pyramid, summarizing the Food and Drug Administration's (FDA) daily nutritional recommendations.

gene therapy   A sophisticated medical procedure that treats a disease by altering the genetic structure of diseased cells.

genetic heart disease   Heart problems related to family history that usually show up in adulthood.

genogram   A schematic representation (drawing) of a family's medical history.

heart transplant   A medical procedure in which a diseased heart is surgically removed and replaced with a heart from a human donor.

hemoglobin   A substance contained in red blood cells that binds with oxygen molecules.

Holter monitor   An ambulatory ECG that can record the heart's activity for 24 hours or longer. Especially helpful for diagnosing transient symptoms (those that come and go without any predictability), such as rhythm problems, atrial fibrillation, and angina. *See also* electrocardiogram (ECG, EKG).

homeocysteine   A toxic waste product produced during cellular metabolism. A high blood homeocysteine level correlates with early, serious heart disease.

homeostasis   The process by which the body adjusts its functions to compensate for deficiencies.

hydrogenation   A process that adds consistency to a product that would otherwise be fairly liquid, such as solid cooking oils and stick margarines. Hydrogenation produces trans–fatty acids (sometimes called trans-fats).

hypertension   The medical term for high blood pressure.

hypotension   The medical term for low blood pressure.

ICD   *Implantable cardioverter defibrillator*. An electronic device implanted into the body that can send brief, regular impulses to the heart to thwart fibrillation, deliver a mild shock to redirect the heart to a normal rhythm (called *cardioversion*), or give a stiff shock to jolt the heart out of a dangerous fibrillation.

imaging procedures   High-tech procedures that let doctors observe various aspects of the heart at work without opening the chest. Includes echocardiography, angiography, CT scan (computerized tomography), and MRI (magnetic resonance imaging). *See also* angiography, echocardiography, MRI, CT scan.

immunosuppressive drugs   Drugs that fool the immune system into accepting a transplanted organ, such as a heart, as if it were native to the host body to prevent rejection.

inspiration   The process by which the lungs take in air; also called *inhalation.*

introvert   A person who processes information internally or inwardly, by thinking about it and mulling it over.

ischemia   Without enough blood (oxygen). Can be myocardial (heart) or brain (transischemic attacks or mini-strokes).

leukocytes   White blood cells.

maximum heart rate   The fastest and hardest your heart can pump without going into fibrillation. Differs according to age.

meditation   A means of focusing the mind to reduce or eliminate conscious thought, to bring the mind to stillness or rest.

metaphysics   A school of philosophical thought that examines the basic nature of reality and existence. The word means "after the physical."

MRI   *Magnetic resonance imaging,* a noninvasive, sophisticated imaging technology using a very strong magnetic field to create images of internal organs.

myocardial infarction   "To block around the heart." Identifies heart tissue that dies because it has been too long without oxygen.

myocardium   A strong, special kind of muscle tissue, not found anywhere else in the body, that makes the heart.

natural selection   The process by which stronger individuals within a species survive and pass their genes to future generations. Weaker individuals are unable to survive and don't reproduce, eliminating their genes from future generations.

naturopathy   A form of alternative medicine that uses substances found naturally in the environment for healing and to maintain health. Also called *naturopathic medicine.*

neuropeptides   Strings of amino acids that carry molecular messages from the brain to the cells.

nicotine   An addictive chemical substance found in tobacco.

noninvasive   Without entering the body.

nutritionist   Someone who has completed a program of study in nutrition or food science. Those who meet the educational and clinical requirements and pass a national test are also registered dietitians, which they designate by placing the initials "RD" after their names.

olestra   A fat-based product with molecules that are too big for the body to digest in the time it takes a product that contains olestra to pass through the digestive system. Used as a fat substitute in snack foods.

omega-3 fatty acids   Special polyunsaturated fats found in fish that keep triglycerides from forming.

organ donor   A person who gives his or her organs for transplant after death.

organ recipient   A person who receives an organ for transplant.

organ rejection   The process by which the immune system perceives a transplanted organ as harmful and attacks it.

pacemaker   An implantable electronic device that regulates the heartbeat.

"pear" body shape   Extra body weight carried through the hips, buttocks, and thighs. Correlates to less of a risk for heart disease than "apple" body shape.

pericardium   The tough sac of fibrous tissue that surrounds the heart and anchors it within the chest.

plaque   The fatty material that builds up on the insides of artery walls.

plasma   The straw-colored fluid component of blood that transports other blood cells and keeps the blood vessels from collapsing.

platelets   Blood cells that contain fibrin (a clotting substance) for repairing wounds.

polyunsaturated fats   Unsaturated fats with many solo (unattached) carbon atoms.

precipitating event   The activity or circumstance that initiates a heart attack, such as sudden physical exertion (like shoveling snow).

primary care physician   An internist (a specialist in adult care) or a family doctor who administers general care.

pulmonary artery   The large artery through which the heart sends blood to the lungs to be oxygenated.

radial artery   The artery felt on the inside of the wrist at the base of the thumb. Often used for taking the pulse.

radionuclides   Radioactive substances injected into the body that release particles of energy. Sophisticated scanning technologies track these particles as they enter various body tissues.

registered dietitian   A nutritionist who meets the educational and clinical requirements and passes a national test. Designated with the initials "RD" after the person's name.

resting pulse rate   How fast and hard the heart beats at rest. Between 70 and 100 for most adults.

saturated fats   Fats that are usually solid at room temperature, such as butter, lard, and animal fat.

sedentary   A lifestyle with very little physical activity.

sinoatrial node   The pea-sized cluster of special-duty cells at the right atrium that generates the tiny jolts of electricity that ripple through the heart muscle to initiate each cardiac cycle.

sphygmomanometer   A device for measuring blood pressure, commonly called a *blood pressure cuff*. Includes an inflatable cuff that wraps around the upper arm, a bulb attached to a tube to pump the cuff full of air, and a gauge that shows the level of pressure within the arteries as the heart beats.

stent   A tiny, spring-like device that keeps an artery's walls from closing again after a coronary bypass graft or balloon angioplasty.

stethoscope   A simple instrument for listening to the heart and lungs.

stroke   Loss of oxygen to the brain caused by a blood clot (ischemic) or bleeding (hemorrhagic).

systole   Means "to contract." The time during which the heart muscle contracts to pump blood out. The higher number in a blood pressure reading.

tachycardia   A heart rate that is faster than normal.

tai chi   An ancient form of martial arts that emphasizes breathing techniques and structured, slow movements. Also incorporates meditation.

target heart rate   The pulse needed to give the heart a good workout. Between 50 and 75 percent of the maximum heart rate.

thrombolytics   Drugs that rapidly dissolve blood clots, "unplugging" blocked arteries to restore blood flow. Sometimes called *clot busters*.

transducer   An electronic device, handheld for most ultrasound procedures, that sends out and receives very high-pitched sound waves (too high for the human ear to detect) for diagnostic imaging.

transischemic attack (TIA)   "Mini-strokes" that occur when a small blood clot blocks an artery leading to the brain for a short time. Symptoms are the same as for a stroke but go away in a few minutes. TIAs often warn that a full-fledged stroke is on the way.

triglyceride   A form of fat closely related to cholesterol.

"ultrafast" CT scan   *Electron beam computed tomography* (EBCT), a sophisticated imaging technology that uses very fast-moving particles to generate clear images of moving organs, such as the heart.

ultrasound   A diagnostic imaging procedure using very high-pitched sound waves to produce pictures of internal organs. Also called *sonography*.

unsaturated fats Fats that are usually liquid at room temperature, sometimes called *oils*.

vascular Having to do with the blood vessels.

vasodilator A drug that causes the arteries to relax so blood can flow through them more easily.

vegetarian A diet that excludes meat so is naturally low in fat. A meatless diet that includes dairy products and some poultry and fish is called *semivegetarian*. A meatless diet that includes milk and eggs, but no fish or poultry, is called *lacto-ovovegetarian*; one that excludes eggs as well is called *lactovegetarian*. A *vegan* diet is the strictest form of vegetarian diet and excludes all animal products, including eggs and dairy.

vena cava Large veins that carry blood into the heart. The *superior vena cava* brings blood from the upper parts of the body. The *inferior vena cava* brings blood from the lower parts of the body.

ventricle The lower, pumping chambers of the heart.

vital signs Blood pressure, pulse, and rate of respiration. Sometimes includes body temperature.

yoga Combines flexibility and breathing techniques to improve physical strength and endurance. Also emphasizes the mind's awareness of the body's activities, connecting body and mind to improve the performance of both.

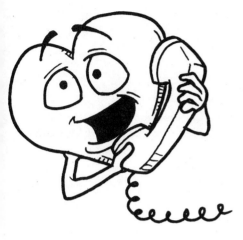

Resources for a Happy, Healthy Heart

American Cancer Society (ACS)
1599 Clifton Road, N.E.
Atlanta, GA 30329
(800) ACS-2345; (404) 320-3333
www.cancer.org

The ACS sponsors support groups and seminars, as well as provides information on the health risks of smoking and how to stop smoking.

American Diabetes Association
1660 Duke Street
Alexandria, VA 22314
(800) 232-3472; (703) 549-1500
www.diabetes.org

Diabetes Forecast, a monthly magazine, and *Diabetes,* a quarterly newsletter, are available to general subscribers, as well as numerous other publications, including a diabetes cookbook series. The association provides counseling, retreats, and other patient-education forums.

American Dietetic Association (ADA)
216 W. Jackson Blvd., Suite 800
Chicago, IL 60606
(312) 899-0040
www.eatright.org

Write or call for a list of cookbooks and other consumer publications on diet and nutrition. Contact the ADA's nutrition hotline, sponsored by its National Center for Nutrition and Dietetics, at (800) 366-1655.

American Heart Association (AHA)
National Center
7320 Greenville Avenue
Dallas, TX 75231
(214) 373-6300
www.americanheart.org

The AHA publishes numerous fact sheets, brochures, and audiovisuals on heart health and heart disease, including many aimed at helping people to reduce their risks. Contacting this organization is a must!

American Institute of Stress
124 Park Avenue
Yonkers, NY 10703
(800) 24-RELAX (247-3529)

Write or call for more information on a variety of stress management techniques from biofeedback to yoga, massage, and meditation.

American Lung Association (ALA)
1740 Broadway
New York, NY 10019
(212) 315-8700
www.lungusa.org

The ALA sponsors seminars and programs on how to quit smoking. It publishes numerous articles and booklets on topics related to the dangers of smoking and nicotine and offers "Freedom from Smoking in 20 Days," a self-help program to stop smoking.

Association for Applied Psychophysiology and Biofeedback
10200 West 44th Avenue, Suite 304
Wheat Ridge, CO 80033
(800) 477-8892

Write or call for information on heart-healthy biofeedback techniques to reduce stress.

Consumer Information Center (CIC)
Pueblo, CO 81009

The CIC catalog features 200 free or low-cost booklets on many topics, including health-related issues such as nutrition, women's health, and smoking. Write for a free copy.

Department of Health and Human Services
www.healthfinder.gov

HHS's user-friendly Web site makes searching for reliable health and human services information easy. There are links on the top health topics, and for every age group, details on health stories in the news. Other sections help you make smart choices about a healthy lifestyle, doctors, healthcare, and health insurance. You'll also find hotlines to report fraud and complaints.

Food and Drug Administration (FDA)
Office of Consumer Affairs, HFE-88
5600 Fishers Lane
Rockville, MD 20857
(301) 443-3170
www.fda.gov

The FDA's monthly journal, *FDA Consumer,* reports on topics of interest to consumers in the regulation of foods, drugs, and cosmetics—including articles on heart bypass surgery and women's nutrition. Subscriptions can be ordered through the Consumer Information Center (see previous listing).

Food and Nutrition Information Center (FNIC)
National Agricultural Library
10301 Baltimore Avenue, Room 304
Beltsville, MD 20705-2351
www.nalusda.gov/fnic

The FNIC performs database searches and provides bibliographies and resource guides on food and nutrition.

Heart Information Network
www.heartinfo.com

HeartInfo is an independent, educational Web site that provides a wide range of information and services to heart patients and others interested in learning about lowering risk factors for heart disease.

Integral Yoga Institute
227 West 13th Street
New York, NY 10011
(212) 929-0586
E-mail: IYI@aol.com

Offers Hatha yoga classes as well as courses in meditation, relaxation, breathing, and yoga for stress management. Also offers a yoga teacher training curriculum.

National Cancer Institute (NCI)
Office of Cancer Communications
Bldg. 31, Room 10A24
9000 Rockville Pike
Bethesda, MD 20892
(800) 4-CANCER; (301) 496-5583
www.nci.nih.gov

NCI publishes and disseminates information about the dangers of smoking and how to quit smoking—including a self-quiz, "Why Do You Smoke?"

National Clearinghouse for Alcohol and Drug Abuse Information (NCADI)
P.O. Box 2345
Rockville, MD 20852
(800) 729-6686; (301) 468-2600
www.health.org

The NCADI has several publications related to the dangers of alcohol and other drugs, including information on topics such as "Alcohol, Tobacco, and Other Drugs May Harm the Unborn."

National Diabetes Information Clearinghouse (NDIC)
Box NDIC
9000 Rockville Pike
Bethesda, MD 20892
(301) 468-2162
www.niddk.nih.gov/health/diabetes/ndic

The NDIC gives information to patients and families about diabetes and its management. The NDIC publishes bibliographies on topics of interest, including diet, nutrition, and pregnancy, as well as a bimonthly newsletter, *Diabetes Dateline.*

National Heart, Lung, and Blood Institute (NHLBI)
Information Center
NHLBI Information Center
P.O. Box 30105
Bethesda, MD 20824-0105
(301) 251-1222
www.nhlbi.nih.gov/nhlbi/nhlbi.htm

The NHLBI, a branch of the National Institutes of Health, sponsors this service providing information about high blood pressure, cholesterol, smoking, obesity, and heart disease. Fact sheets on topics related to heart health and disease are also available. Write or call for a directory of publications.

National Library of Medicine
U.S. Department of Health and Human Services
Building 38A, Room 3N-305
8600 Rockville Pike
Bethesda, MD 20894
(301) 496-1131

Write or call to order a free directory of health-related organizations with 800 numbers nationwide.

National Stroke Association (NSA)
96 Inverness Drive East, Suite I
Englewood, CO 80112
(303) 649-9299
www.stroke.org

The NSA is the only national voluntary healthcare organization that focuses 100 percent of its resources and attention on stroke prevention, treatment, rehabilitation, research, and support for stroke survivors and their families.

Office of Disease Prevention and Health Promotion
National Health Information Center (ONHIC)
P.O. Box 1133
Washington, DC 20013-1133
(800) 336-4797; (301) 565-4167
odphp.oash.dhhs.gov

The ONHIC provides laypeople and healthcare professionals with pathways to research health topics of interest through its information and referral system and resource guides. Write for a listing of publications.

Stress Reduction Clinic
University of Massachusetts Medical Center
55 Lake Avenue, North
Worcester, MA 01655
(508) 856-2656

Founded and directed by Dr. Jon Kabat-Zinn, the author of several best-selling books on stress reduction and mindfulness meditation, the Stress Reduction Clinic at the University of Massachusetts Medical Center is renowned for its work with patients who have chronic illnesses. Stress reduction video and audiotapes can be ordered from the clinic by direct mail.

U.S. Government Printing Office
Superintendent of Documents
Washington, DC 20402-9352
(202) 783-3238

Write for a free copy of "U.S. Government Books and New Books."

Index

A

G - H